BLACK
HEALTH
MATTERS

THE VITAL FACTS YOU MUST KNOW TO PROTECT
YOUR HEALTH AND THAT OF YOUR LOVED ONES

RICHARD W. WALKER, JR., MD

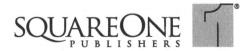
SQUAREONE
PUBLISHERS

The information and advice contained in this book are based upon the research and the personal and professional experiences of the author. They are not intended as a substitute for consulting with a health care professional. The publisher and author are not responsible for any adverse effects or consequences resulting from the use of any of the suggestions discussed in this book. All matters pertaining to your physical health should be supervised by a health care professional. It is a sign of wisdom, not cowardice, to seek a second or third opinion.

COVER DESIGNER: Jeannie Rosado
EDITOR: Joanne Abrams
TYPESETTER: Gary A. Rosenberg

Square One Publishers
115 Herricks Road
Garden City Park, NY 11040
(516) 535-2010 • (877) 900-BOOK
www.squareonepublishers.com

Library of Congress Cataloging-in-Publication Data
Names: Walker, Richard W., Jr., author.
Title: Black health matters : the vital facts you must know to protect your
   health and that of your loved ones / Richard W. Walker, Jr., MD.
Description: Garden City Park : Square One Publishers, [2021] | Includes
   bibliographical references and index
Identifiers: LCCN 2021020057 (print) | LCCN 2021020058 (ebook) | ISBN
   9780757005077 (paperback) | ISBN 9780757055072 (ebook)
Subjects: LCSH: African Americans--Health and hygiene.
Classification: LCC RA448.5.N4 W37 2021 (print) | LCC RA448.5.N4 (ebook)
   | DDC 613.089/96073--dc23
LC record available at https://lccn.loc.gov/2021020057
LC ebook record available at https://lccn.loc.gov/2021020058

To my best friend and wife, Marvia.
There would be no *Black Health Matters*,
nor any "Richard W. Walker, Jr. MD," without you.
Thank you for your life with me.

Contents

Acknowledgments

No book of this scope can be put together without help. I want to thank Carol Nicholson for her wisdom and inspiration in telling me, "You should write a book and title it *Black Health Matters.*" I am also grateful to Sonia Dunbar, a superb geriatric dental hygienist—AKA, "The Geriatric Tooth Fairy"—for writing the chapter on oral health. I learned more from her about oral healthcare than I did in all of medical school. And special thanks to Laura Stevens, the author of many health publications, for helping me with the overall writing of this book.

I must also thank Joanne Abrams, the book's editor, who did a masterful job. And, of course, Rudy Shur, CEO of Square One Publishers. I call Rudy "the Principal," like the school principal, as I was always in his "email office." The expression "iron sharpens iron" applies here, because Rudy and I would go at it, back and forth, on nearly every aspect of this book, trying to make certain it had just enough science, enough energy, and enough "readability" to enable people to understand it and finish it. Rudy would say, "Let's make this book as good as it can be." I hope we have.

However, in order to write this book, I had to start where everything begins. This book is about helping others, so it's about being a servant. Therefore, I must begin by acknowledging my Lord Jesus Christ, who gave me the wherewithal to get here, and my parents, Richard and Ellena, who made certain I always studied in school and didn't hang out in the streets of Spanish Harlem.

I also give my thanks to USAF Major Raymond Sumners (Ret.), a white man who taught me how to navigate and be successful in the military despite being confronted by major discrimination. He taught me all the instrumentation and techniques of being a lab tech at the USAF's Epidemiological Laboratory at Lackland Air Force Base in Texas. He held nothing back. Also to the late Professor and Dean Alexander Joseph, PhD, of the Department of Science and Forensic Science at John Jay College of Criminal Justice, who forced me to apply to medical school because, as he said, "I see something in you." And to Clarence Porter, MD, my longtime friend and colleague who made significant contributions to the direction of my career and life. Now he's my partner and co-founder of our healthcare company, Walker Health Care Holdings, Inc., and TVP-Care.

And then there is my best friend and wife, Marvia, who always had the right words at the right time and never hesitated to navigate the paths taken, both known and unknown, no matter the difficulty or the circumstance. She is how I know God exists. Because of Marvia, we have our own cheerleading team, mob, crew, bunch—our children, Carmen and Mark, and their spouses, Darrell and Rosa. They produced the rest of the bunch, with everyone cheering Marvia ("Schranny," as the grandkids call her) and me on in everything we do. Our children and their spouses use conservative cheerleading language: "You can do it." But our grandchildren—Jamila ("Milzy"), the oldest, a world traveler, chef, and entrepreneur; Samantha ("Z"), full of energy and excitement, and a University of Michigan sophomore (my alma mater); Jada and Spencer, ninth-grade cousins born twenty-four hours apart, and both characters and opposites; and Leena, a seventh grader very much like her grandmother, quiet but very aware and observant—are the ultimate reasons for this book and the ultimate cheerleaders. They do not hold back, telling me to "do it" with exuberance, as well as facial and body expressions that reflect their generation. The best part is that whenever I tell them what I have done, they know that there's nothing that they can't do.

Preface

I was raised in Spanish Harlem during the 1950s and 1960s, where I saw firsthand the men in my friends' families and my own family simply disappear from the community. I didn't understand why that was happening. Looking back, and after speaking to many of my friends over the years, I discovered that most of the men disappeared for multiple reasons, all of which were tragic. I was simply too young to understand the devastating social and racial reasons why this was taking place. So many suffered from severe high blood pressure resulting in strokes, heart attacks, kidney failure, and eventually death. Diabetes was the real scourge, causing wholesale amputations and blindness. Diabetes terrified me and everyone else, because it was a complete mystery, like a ghost that could come and get you at any time. And none of these men was taking medications to control their health disorders. They went to the doctor only after a catastrophe, and by then, it was too late.

The plight of the men in my community made me angry, but it seemed too late for me to do anything to help them. However, after serving for four years in the US Air Force, as a Vietnam-era veteran, I was able to focus on my education and my future. I enrolled at John Jay College and graduated in 1974. I then had the opportunity to go to the Albert Einstein College of Medicine. I did my residency training in Obstetrics and Gynecology at the University of Michigan, and I practiced for twenty years. But over time, I became dissatisfied with traditional medicine, which focused on treating illness rather than maintaining wellness. I therefore went back to school to study STD Epidemiology at Johns Hopkins, Environmental Medicine at the SW Naturopathic College, Age Management Medicine at the Cenegenics Institute, and Functional Medicine at the Institute for Functional Medicine, becoming certified in all. These schools teach people how to take control of their own health.

After two decades of practicing traditional medicine, I practiced Environmental and Functional Medicine for the next fifteen years. For several years, I also had my own radio talk show in New York City, where the topics were anything but conventional. Instead, whether I was addressing my patients or my radio audience, I provided information about wellness through nutrition, supplements, nutraceuticals (foods or food components that provide medical or health benefits), and Environmental and Age Management Medicine. My goal was to tell people how they could avoid the misery of chronic illness by taking responsibility for their own health. It was important information for everyone, but I always tried to provide information that was especially relevant to Black communities.

Through proper diet, exercise, and other lifestyle changes, as well as the use of selected nutritional supplements, they could maintain good health for much of their lives. And if a health condition did occur, they could manage it better if they relied not just on standard medicine—although standard medicine might be necessary—but also on healthy lifestyle practices. In other words, instead of depending on the medical community to deal with their diseases, they would make the medical community a partner, and the emphasis would be on prevention rather than treatment.

In my practice, I could see that my approach to wellness worked. But so many people in Black communities were still suffering from chronic illness because they didn't know that there was a better way, and I didn't know how to reach them all. Then in 2020—in the middle of the pandemic that hit the Black community especially hard—something happened. After the brutal death of George Floyd, the mantra of "Black Lives Matter" became prominent in the American lexicon. One day, a friend and nurse, Carol Nicholson, called and simply said, "You should write a book and title it *Black*

Health Matters." It was an epiphany. Here was an opportunity to do something about my lingering concerns over the perennial Black health condition and perhaps reach many thousands of people in the process.

Thus, I began my work on the book you now hold in your hands. Naturally, *Black Health Matters* reflects my training as a doctor in all its components—particularly in Environmental and Functional Medicine—with the goal of improving the health and wellness of African Americans and their families. But *Black Health Matters* also reflects my continuing research into the cause of disease—both in the Black community and in the larger community—and into the many ways in which individuals can avoid and/or manage disease through lifestyle choices that are entirely within their control. Because I think that every individual should have access to this research, for each chapter, you'll find a list of the sources I have used in the References section.

In this book, I have tried to address all of the main chronic health problems that affect African Americans: obesity, hypertension, diabetes, cardiovascular disease, kidney disease, and dental disease, as well as sickle cell disease. I also examine important issues such as aging, environmental health, and healthcare and racism. Since so many chronic illnesses have been caused in large part by poor food choices, a separate chapter is devoted to nutrition and diets. This chapter will help you not only select better foods but also use diet to prevent and manage illness. Each chapter of the book builds upon the others, providing secrets and opportunities to improve your well-being.

As you read through the chapters on different common disorders and problems, you may find certain issues being discussed in more than one chapter. In the paragraph above, I mention that a good diet is vital in the avoidance and treatment of every condition mentioned in this book. Other lifestyle-related behaviors, like exercise, are also crucial as you strive for better health, as is the use of dietary supplements such as vitamin D_3. This is why you will see these issues discussed several times within the pages of the book.

Throughout my medical career, Black patients have told me about their family's genetic predisposition to chronic disease. But if we accept the idea that we are genetically predestined to get these diseases we face as a people, there's no hope. This book was written to tell you that this idea is at worst a lie, and at best, just plain wrong. You can take control and live a longer, healthier life. *Black Health Matters* can show you how it's done.

Introduction

"I am no longer accepting the things I cannot change.
I am changing the things I can no longer accept."
—DR. ANGELA DAVIS

Black Health Matters was written with a single purpose—to empower you, the reader, to take control of your own health and healthcare. This means positioning yourself to make informed decisions about your well-being and that of your loved ones. Of course, you need to work with your healthcare professional, but to accomplish this, you must be armed with knowledge and understanding. Every day, you have to remain in control of your lifestyle and the decisions that will affect your health. To achieve this, you need a blueprint for improving your health and maintaining it. That is what *Black Health Matters* is all about.

It is easy enough to say "Black health matters." But when we go by the numbers, the extent of poor health among our Black population becomes painfully evident. According to the Centers for Disease Control (CDC), health disparities continue to exist due to poverty, unequal access to care, and unequal representation in medical research. That painful truth was just as evident to Martin Luther King, Jr., when he said, "Of all the forms of inequality, injustice in health is the most shocking and the most inhuman because it often results in physical death." However, we have to understand that this inequality goes back hundreds of years.

BLACK HEALTHCARE VERSUS WHITE HEALTHCARE

Throughout American history, healthcare for White Americans has always been shamefully better than that for Black Americans, contributing to a greater number of Blacks with chronic illness and early deaths. If you take the same chronic diseases that White Americans die from as seniors—that is, at sixty-five-plus years— you will find Black Americans dying of these conditions in their twenties, thirties, and forties. That is because, as a group, Black Americans get chronic diseases earlier in life than White Americans, and this earlier onset leads to disabilities and earlier deaths. Unfortunately, there are many reasons for this.

Cost

Since costs and/or the lack of health insurance determines if you see a doctor early and often, it is, without a doubt, a major contributor to the problem now faced by African Americans. First, let's look at the inequality in healthcare insurance. Coverage by health insurance for Blacks at all ages has been persistently lower than that for Whites. Many hourly jobs that Blacks hold do not include health insurance, and lack of coverage is a barrier for receiving health services. The cost of insurance is higher for Blacks than for Whites, and if you don't have health insurance, a doctor may require substantially higher payments to see and treat you.

After the Affordable Care Act (ACA) was passed in 2014, more Blacks Americans had insurance coverage. However, 30 million people, half of them persons of color, remained uninsured in the United States. Fourteen states, mostly in the South, refused to expand Medicaid, depriving many Blacks of coverage. Medicaid coverage is crucial for elderly and underserved Blacks. However, it still does not pay the full cost of hospital stays and doctor's visits, nor does it fully cover prescription drugs. Furthermore, many doctors will not accept patients who have Medicaid because it pays them peanuts, if they get paid at all. Out-of-pocket costs are a burden for recipients with low incomes and high healthcare needs.

The Lack of Local Medical Facilities

In some cases, adequate medical facilities may be far away from Black communities, especially in rural areas. Added to that is the lack of transportation to the medical facility due to high costs or the lack of routes in neighborhoods. Too often, in urban communities, the only option for immediate healthcare may be a visit to a hospital emergency room, which becomes their main source of healthcare. And once there, a patient may likely wait hours to be seen.

The harsh reality is that many of these medical care centers and doctors' offices avoid opening in poorer communities because of economic reasons or perceived safety concerns. And while this great divide of medical care may not have been based on racism or ethnicity, it has excluded poorer communities from getting essential services.

Keeping Appointments

For Black hourly workers, keeping a healthcare appointment during a work day is often discouraged or even disallowed by many employers. This is due to the long time it takes to see a doctor. In fact, the average wait time for Black folks is roughly seventy minutes versus fifty-three minutes for Whites. Try explaining that to an employer when you are two or three hours late. And even when workers try to get an appointment before work begins or after it ends, they need to be fitted into the doctor's schedule—which may require weeks or even months of waiting. Too often, the result of these negative experiences is to simply avoid seeing a doctor.

What occurs is a snowballing effect. The delay in seeing the doctor allows the health condition to get worse, which means more time needed for follow-up appointments, which means more absences from work. Then, as all this is occurring, the cost of the care increases due to the frequency of visits and probably more medications. This, in turn, means there may not be enough money to pay the extra costs involved, so patients don't get their appointments completed. This results in the condition progressing from a slowly evolving disease to an immediate and severe condition requiring attention in the Emergency Department, often leading to hospital admissions. Too often this becomes a dangerous cycle.

Poorer Quality of Healthcare

Black people are simply not receiving the fair and impartial healthcare that their White counterparts receive. Even if health insurance, income, age, and severity of conditions are equal to a similar group of Whites, Black care is inferior. The American Bar Association has reported that minority persons are less likely than White persons to receive appropriate cardiac care; kidney dialysis or transplants; and the best treatments for stroke, cancer, or AIDS. Further, the report concluded that conscious or unconscious racism by the doctors plays a role.

COVID-19: A CASE IN POINT

The racial inequities of the healthcare system—and of American society in general—was highlighted by the COVID-19 pandemic, a global pandemic that began in 2019. Communities of color bore the brunt of the pandemic because of higher-risk work environments, crowded urban living conditions, and a higher rate of preexisting conditions. In fact, African American and Latinos were three times more likely than Whites to contract COVID-19. People of color also found it harder to find testing, receive adequate treatment, and—when vaccines became available—to access them. This led to a higher rate of Black and Latino deaths.

For instance, in Louisiana, Blacks represented about one-third of the state population but 70 percent of COVID-19 deaths. At the national level, Pacific Islander, Latino, Indigenous, and Black Americans had a COVID-19 death rate of *double* or more that of Whites and Asian Americans. As Kim Blankenship, Professor of Sociology at American University, said, this is "the price we pay for inequality." Never has the need for societal change been clearer.

Higher Incidence of Chronic Disease

Blacks are at much higher risk for many chronic diseases, yet their ability to have them monitored is far less than Whites. For example, hypertension affects 75 percent of Blacks compared with 55 percent of White men and 40 percent of White women. Hypertension occurs earlier in life for Blacks. Even African American children have higher blood pressure than White children. For the Black community to receive help with this common disorder, their hypertension must be diagnosed early, and their blood pressure monitored regularly by their doctor and themselves. If they receive this diagnosis, their doctor may prescribe blood pressure medicine that effectively lowers blood pressure. While many relatively cheaper drugs are available, drugs are only part of the solution. Patients must understand that they can dramatically lower their blood pressure by lowering their salt intake, losing weight, and exercising. These lifestyle changes rest on the patient's shoulders.

Like hypertension, obesity and type 2 diabetes also affect many more Blacks than Whites. These chronic diseases need to be controlled or eliminated, requiring the input of doctors and their guidance for life-changing efforts. Again, your doctor can only do so much. Much rests on you, the patient.

Inherited Illnesses

Various ethnicities are predisposed to certain conditions. Blacks are genetically more at risk than Whites for some diseases, such as sickle cell disease (SCD), a devastating illness for many Black Americans. In fact, one baby in every 365 Black people is born with SCD. I will talk more about this disease in Chapter 11. However, for the most part, chronic health conditions experienced by African Americans are more strongly related to obesity and poor diet than to genetics.

Poor Diets

Poor diet—due to bad food choices, poverty, and unhealthy eating traditions (sorry)—are major contributing factors in all the chronic diseases that plague Blacks more than Whites. And while processed foods that are high in sugars, "bad" fats, and salt may taste good, they lack basic nutrients—the very cause of so many of the common illnesses we suffer.

In many areas of the United States, Black neighborhoods lack major grocery store chains. Instead, local food shops (bodegas) offer lots of expensive processed foods with no fresh fruits and vegetables and whole grains. Some Blacks cannot afford healthier foods. But if you don't feed your brain and body well, over time, you are likely to develop a chronic illness. With help from this book, you will learn the components of a good diet and avoid the "junk" foods that are all too common in our communities. There's more about this in Chapters 2 and 9.

LIVING HEALTHIER

If you adopt a healthier lifestyle, you may be able to lessen or eliminate the need for chronic healthcare interventions such as medications. Let's be clear about what I mean: I am *not* saying that you should avoid seeing your physician, getting annual exams, and taking prescribed medications. To the contrary, it's essential to get blood work, mammograms, pap smears, prostate exams, regular annual checkups, etc. However, it's also important to stop doing those things that are drivers of ill health. Type 2 diabetes doesn't have to be. Severe hypertension doesn't have to be. Most of all, being overweight or obese doesn't have to be. What you will read repeatedly is that obesity is a gateway disease, meaning that with this condition come most of the other chronic diseases we see in the Black community.

There are basic actions you should take to ensure that your body becomes as healthy as God meant it to be! First, eat a nutritious diet that provides the proper amounts of protein, carbohydrates, fiber, "good" fats, and, perhaps, supplements of vitamins, minerals, essential fatty acids, and other nutrients, depending on your unique health needs. You will also need to exercise and get adequate sleep. It is crucial to reduce the stress in your life—just being Black in America is stressful! Learn to relax, perhaps by walking, taking up yoga or tai chi, or listening to calming music. If you want to achieve good health, all these things are critical for your success. As a bonus, when you start feeling better, you may feel less stressed.

On the other hand, to achieve good health, you must change some harmful behaviors. If you are overweight or obese, you need to eat less. Also avoid processed foods that are loaded with white flour, too many calories, too much salt, excessive sugar and corn syrup, "bad" fats, and artificial chemicals. The latter are added by manufacturers to deceive you, the consumer. Don't play their game! They are just out to make more money by selling nutritionally empty foods that are cheap to manufacture.

Second, you must decrease your indoor and outdoor exposure to toxic chemicals, because these substances can make you sick. If you smoke, you must stop. You already know that, and on numerous occasions, you may have promised yourself and others to kick the habit. This time, you need to follow through. Constant exposure to poor foods and harmful chemicals will eventually mean that your body stops working properly, causing an early development of chronic disease and an untimely death.

You must take advantage of today's technology to learn as much as you can about your health and how to change it. Then you need to act on that knowledge. You cannot be ignorant of currently available information and then say, "The devil made me do it" or "I can hardly move because I weigh too much, but I just love food! I can't stop myself!" That is a myth, and the continued belief that the problem is someone else's fault, that change is someone else's responsibility, or that change is just too difficult will keep you from reaching your goal of better health and a better life.

WHAT'S TO COME

In the following chapters, I will share the knowledge you need to improve your health and I will outline the steps you must take. You will need to find a healthcare practitioner to assess your health, monitor your progress, prescribe vital medications, and, hopefully, cheer you on. With his or her input, you must also take control of your own health. How do you that? Reading the following chapters should be a good start.

Chapter 1 discusses the microscopic organisms that populate your gut. I know it's hard to believe, but there are trillions of these one-celled organisms! When they are in balance, your body works well, but when they get out of balance, your health suffers. This chapter introduces you to the microbiome—the community of microbes (bacteria, more commonly known as germs) in your body—and aids you in keeping that community healthy.

The obesity epidemic is sweeping this country. Obesity contributes to heart disease, stroke, type 2 diabetes, and some cancers. Blacks, especially Black women, are more likely to be overweight, obese, and even morbidly obese than Whites. Chapter 2 discusses the problem of obesity and provides the steps you can take to achieve a thinner you.

Chapter 3 discusses another epidemic: hypertension. Hypertension, or high blood pressure, is a silent killer. It doesn't have symptoms to warn you to get medical help, and it is associated with many serious disorders. In this chapter, you will learn why hypertension is so dangerous, what causes it, and how you can lower your risks of getting this insidious disease.

Diabetes is a major public health problem that is approaching epidemic proportions globally, and is found in high numbers in the African-American community. Chapter 4 takes a close look at this disorder—its causes, its diagnosis, and its complications. Most important, it tells you the many simple steps you can take to lower your risk or, if you already have diabetes, to help control it.

Cardiovascular disease consistently remains the leading cause of death in the United States. Worse still, nearly 48 percent of Black women and 44 percent of Black men have some form of this disease. Chapter 5 explains what cardiovascular disease is, what causes it, and what you can do—from improving your diet to exercising—to avoid heart disease, heart attack, and stroke.

Statistics show that Black Americans are four times more likely to fall victim to kidney disease than White Americans—even though Blacks make up only about 13 percent of the population. Chapter 6 explores the many risk factors associated with kidney disease, explains how it is connected to other disorders that plague the Black community, and lists its early symptoms so that you can help identify this problem and stop it in its tracks.

Although the overall cancer death rates have dropped faster in Blacks than in Whites, African Americans with cancer still have the shortest survival rates of any racial and ethnic group in the country. Fortunately, there are many things you can do to protect yourself and your loved ones from this terrible disease. Chapter 7 starts by explaining what cancer is. It then discusses the many causes of cancer and, most important, the ways in which you can reduce your risk.

The focus of Chapter 8 is the issue of aging. Although no one can stay young forever, it is possible to get older without being disabled by age-related disorders, and it's also possible to lengthen your life span. This chapter first explains how the natural process of aging affects the body. It then shows you that by making simple lifestyle changes and taking selected supplements, you can live longer and, just as important, live healthier.

In almost every chapter of this book, we highlight how good nutrition can help you avoid or better manage many common health disorders. Chapter 9 focuses on this issue, telling you everything you need to know to improve your diet and your health. You'll first learn about the history of Black nutrition in America, see why our communities eat the way they do, and understand how this impacts our health. The chapter then guides you in choosing nutritious foods—vegetables, fruits, whole grains, lean proteins, beans, nuts, dairy products, and other foods that if prepared properly can help you avoid all those nasty disorders discussed throughout this book. Following this, you discover how specific diets—including the American Heart Association Diet, Mediterranean Diet, DASH Diet, and vegetarian diets—can help treat specific medical conditions, such as obesity and hypertension, as well as improve your overall well-being. Finally, Chapter 9 examines fasting, which many people successfully use to lose weight, detoxify their cells, lower blood pressure, and provide many other benefits. Throughout, you'll learn interesting information about probiotic foods, complex carbohydrates, flavonoids, and other foods and food components that can make your body the best it can be.

Chapter 10 is all about your environment, including the apartment or house where you live, your neighborhood, your children's schools, and your work place. For decades, if not centuries, Black communities have suffered from some of the most harmful environments in the United States. This chapter looks at how the environment profoundly affects our health, and examines the specific substances—such as asbestos, lead, mold, and plastics—that are harming us and our children. Finally, it suggests practical changes you can make to improve the quality of your air, remove toxins from your diet, and detoxify your body. Just as important, it urges you to demand actions that would improve the environment of Black communities.

Chapter 11 tackles the problem of sickle cell disease (SCD), a genetic disorder that plagues the Black community, causing an endless list of problems, such as severe pain, frequent infection, vision problems, and organ damage. After explaining sickle cell disease and its effects on the body, this chapter discusses testing, symptoms and complications, and standard treatments. Finally, it explores two cutting-edge procedures that show great promise in the treatment of SCD, and in some cases, may even eliminate the disease.

In Chapter 12, you will learn about common dental and oral problems and explore how poor dental health can affect your overall health—how, amazingly, it can even damage the heart, the kidneys, blood sugar levels, blood pressure, and more. Unfortunately, Black communities usually have little access to good affordable dental care. This chapter provides tips for improving your oral health on your own and also offers practical suggestions for finding a good reasonably priced dentist in your area.

The Conclusion takes a hard look at healthcare, race, and racial disparities in the healthcare system. It examines long-standing racial disparities in our nation's healthcare and looks at this pivotal moment in our country, when African Americans must not only take responsibility for their own health but also call for change in the way they are treated by medical professionals.

Before you begin reading the chapters on specific disorders, such as hypertension and diabetes, I want you to understand that although I sometimes touch on the standard medical treatments that are used in the management of these disorders, that is not my focus in this book. Although medication is necessary to treat certain ailments, I have learned in my practice that it is often possible to avoid these illnesses or manage them with less medication if the individual is willing to modify diet, increase exercise, and make other lifestyle changes.

With that being said, I want to caution you that if you are using medications prescribed for you by your doctor, you should not stop taking these drugs—even if you feel that your health has improved—without contacting your physician and determining if it would be safe to do so. Similarly, if you are being treated for a medical condition, you should not begin taking nutritional supplements before discussing the specifics with your health-care provider. Some supplements interact poorly with certain medications.

Following the Conclusion of *Black Health Matters*, you will find a wealth of material that can help you better understand the issues discussed in this book and take the first step towards better health. The Glossary explains many of the terms used in the book that may be new to you. The Guide to Dietary Supplements provides important information about choosing and using supplements, and recommends the best nutrients for treating the diseases covered in the book. A Resources section guides you to organizations, websites, books, and other resources that can provide you with further information about diet, environmental toxins, and much more. And if you're interested in looking at the studies and articles on which this book was based, you can turn to the References section.

Throughout the book I have included Black health Timelines. All too often, we hear stories about the exploitation of Blacks throughout history. Rarely do we learn about how our community has endured years of suffering due to medical mistreatment and abuse. We are where we are because of this history. While I have made the stories brief, each one is telling. As survivors, we must learn from the past so that we never have to repeat it.

CONCLUSION

I understand that many African-American families have achieved a level of economic success, giving them access to better health-care. That being said, they are just as susceptible to each and every health issue discussed in this book. This is why *Black Health Matters* is designed to help every Black person achieve better health, just as I have successfully guided my own patients to greater well-being during my many years as a practicing physician. By following the advice offered in this book, you can turn your life around, feel better—perhaps better than you have in a long time—and enjoy many happy, healthy years to come.

1

The Gut-Microbiome-Brain Connection

"Lots of people think, well, we're humans; we're the most intelligent and accomplished species; we're in charge. Bacteria may have a different outlook: more bacteria live and work in one linear centimeter of your lower colon than all the humans who have ever lived. That's what's going on in your digestive tract right now. Are we in charge, or are we simply hosts for bacteria? It all depends on your outlook."
—Neil deGrasse Tyson

The Gut-Microbiome-Brain Connection—"What is that?," you might ask. As you will see, it is an early warning system that is responsible for your current state of health, your mental attitude, and all the functions that occur in your body to keep you alive. Most people are unaware of its existence, but it is essential both physiologically and mentally, and in a number of ways, it can even determine life and death. By the time you finish reading this chapter, you will have a better understanding of how this connection plays a vital role in all of the issues discussed in the chapters that follow.

To understand what the Gut-Microbiome-Brain (GMB) Connection is, let's compare the human body to the body of a car. When a car is assembled, it has an engine that will provide it with the power it needs to move from one place to another. It has on-board computers that will connect you to the Internet, tell you if any parts of the car are experiencing problems, and perhaps even allow the car to drive itself. However, none of these functions can work without the use of electricity, oil, and the right fuel. These are the materials that allow the car to do what it was built to do.

In the same way a car is built, your body is "constructed" in your mother's womb. Initially, your working parts are based on the genetics you inherited from your parents, and while in the womb, you are dependent on your mother for everything you need to maintain life and to properly develop—nutrition, oxygen, and antibodies (for future disease prevention)—just as a car depends on gas, oil, and electricity. But on the day of your birth, you are no longer dependent on your mother's direct connection to you through the placenta and umbilical cord. Everything she used to provide directly, you now have to obtain by eating, drinking, and breathing. When you enter this world, you have all the body parts you are going to have for the rest of your life. In addition, you have the GMB Connection, which will enable those parts to work properly.

WHAT IS THE GUT-MICROBIOME-BRAIN (GMB) CONNECTION?

Every metabolic function and chemical reaction in the body—and, therefore, the health of every organ—is directly or indirectly dependent on the proper function of the GMB Connection. When the GMB is disrupted, it's likely to create a problem with your health. To better understand how the GMB works, let's look at each of its parts.

The Gut

Your *gut* is a general name for your gastrointestinal tract. Also referred to as the GI tract, it begins at the mouth and includes all of the organs involved in the digestion and absorption of foods— the mouth, esophagus, stomach, small and large intestines, anus, liver, gall bladder, and pancreas. Each organ has a specific role in keeping you healthy. The ultimate function of the GI system is to break down foods and allow the nutrients to be distributed and used throughout the body to provide the energy and protection you need to survive.

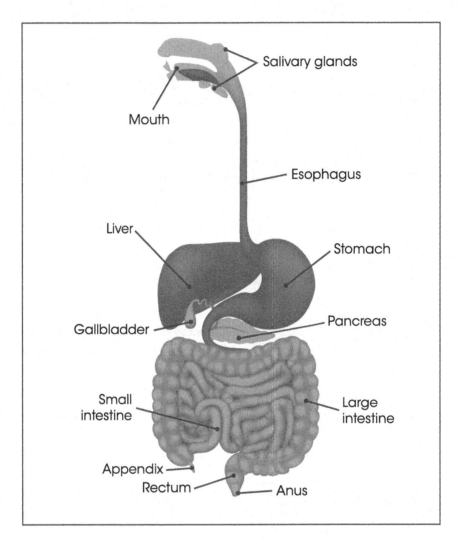

Figure 1.1. The Gut.

The Microbiome

Within your GI tract there exists a world of various tiny microbes, each with its own set of genes. This world is called the *microbiome.* You have your initial exposure to these bacteria during birth as you pass through your mom's birth canal and make contact with vaginal bacteria through your mouth and skin. As a baby, your GI system has the specific bacteria your mom had in her vagina.

These microbes include many different types of bacteria, which vary in number. While bacteria are found throughout the GI tract, the highest concentration is found in the large intestine.

When all of the trillions of microbes in the GI tract are added together, your microbiome may weigh as much as five pounds. In fact, your body contains about ten times more microbial cells than it does human cells. Although these bacteria are single-celled organisms, research shows that they carry out vital tasks throughout your body. The human body's microbes:

● Generate nutrition for human cells by breaking down foods into the basic components—starches, fats, sugars, and proteins—needed to keep the cells alive.

● Synthesize vitamins, including some B vitamins and also vitamin K, which helps your blood clot.

● Regulate your metabolism—the process of converting what you eat into smaller basic building blocks (amino acids, glucose, fatty acids, etc.) while creating energy. These building blocks are then used to create the new proteins, carbohydrates, and fats needed to sustain life.

● Contribute to detoxifying or neutralizing many cancer-causing substances, making them harmless.

● Help renew the growth of cells in the gut lining. This lining is critical for your health because it controls which substances are absorbed and which are not.

● Support the immune system, activating and regulating the immune response.

● Play a significant role in controlling your weight and the development of obesity.

● Create neurotransmitters—chemical messengers such as serotonin—which facilitate communication between the gut and brain as well as other cells in the body.

THE PROS AND CONS OF ANTIBIOTICS

Antibiotics are drugs, such as penicillin, that are designed to kill or inhibit harmful bacteria that enter the body and cause infection. The interesting thing about antibiotics is that they can be both a blessing and a curse. How is this possible? First, antibiotics have saved countless lives by killing harmful bacteria. If you have ever had a bacterial infection such as pneumonia, a urinary tract infection, or strep throat, it was most likely due to harmful bacteria and was treated with an antibiotic. If the antibiotic restored your health, it was definitely a blessing.

On the other hand, antibiotics can also kill many of the good bacteria in your intestine, greatly disturbing the balance of your microbiome. This imbalance—the "curse" referred to earlier—can result in digestive problems such as gas, diarrhea, constipation, heartburn, and more. Fortunately, by taking probiotic supplements, you can help repopulate your microbiome with good bacteria. So if your doctor hands you a prescription for an antibiotic, ask if a probiotic also may be helpful. (See page 23 for more information on probiotics.)

While antibiotics can help restore health in cases of bacterial infection, it is important to note that these drugs cannot be used to treat viral infections or infections caused by fungi or most parasites. When people get a common cold or a case of the flu, they often ask their doctor for antibiotics. Because both influenza and the common cold are viral infections, antibiotics won't work. Additionally, the overuse of antibiotics makes some harmful bacteria resistant to these drugs. Then, when you really need an antibiotic, it may not be helpful. Antibiotic resistance is a huge public health crisis today. This is why antibiotics should be restricted to the treatment of bacterial infections and should be used with care.

When you read about all the vital roles that bacteria play in your body, it becomes clear that when your microbes are out of balance, your body is out of balance. Because your microbiome is dependent on the health and nutrition of your mother when she was pregnant with you, your DNA, your own food choices, the environment in which you live, and even the medications you take (see the inset on page 17), you have a unique set of bacteria, different from everyone else's.

The Brain

As you know, your brain enables you to think, talk, feel, see, hear, remember, walk, and so much more. It also automatically controls your breathing, heartbeat, blinking, and many other vital activities. The brain is a soft mass of more than eighty billion cells called *neurons*, which interconnect with neighboring brain cells to carry messages in the form of electrical impulses from one neuron to the next. An amazing network of blood vessels delivers "food" to the neurons and removes wastes.

The brain is divided into several sections, each of which controls a different function. For the most part, the right side of your brain controls the left side of your body, and the left side of your brain controls the right side of your body. The brain is covered by a layer of specialized cells that form the *blood-brain barrier*, which screens out substances that would disrupt brain function. Finally, the skull encloses the brain and protects it from physical danger.

The Glands

Although the term Gut-Microbiome-Brain Connection does not seem to refer to the body's glands, these organs are vital in connecting the brain to functions throughout the body. Your body has two type of glands, the exocrine glands and the endocrine glands. The *exocrine glands* release substances through ducts that are connected to the outside layer of your body. They are responsible for sweat, saliva, tears, and mother's milk, and thus help regulate body temperature, help protect the eyes, defend against bad bacteria by producing mucus, and nourish babies through breast milk. What they do not do is produce hormones. That is the job of the endocrine glands, and it is these glands that are most critical to the GMB Connection.

STRESS AND THE ADRENAL GLANDS

As you will learn on page 20, the endocrine glands play an important role in functions that take place throughout the body. In the case of the adrenal glands and the hypothalamus, they are responsible for both our short- and long-term management of physical and emotional stress.

There are two adrenal glands, one atop of each kidney. These glands have several functions, one of which is facilitating the body's "flight or fight" response to extremely stressful situations. When the caveman experienced stress, his adrenal glands secreted more of the hormone adrenalin, which increased blood pressure, made his heart beat faster, and caused his body to secrete more insulin, thereby boosting blood sugar levels. This gave him the energy he needed to run for his life when facing a physical threat such as a tiger. After escaping from the tiger, the caveman's hormone levels—and their effects—would return to normal.

Now, just as in the caveman's time, whenever you experience a threat, the gut and brain communicate with each other to create a "gut reaction." You may feel queasy or sick to your stomach. Your heart may race, and you may feel a surge of energy as your body prepares to combat or flee the danger. This is the GMB at work. In today's world, you usually don't have tigers chasing you, but you may have stress resulting from financial problems, job pressures, poor health, and racial discrimination. Something as simple as being pulled over by the police while driving can trigger great stress.

Since stresses in the twenty-first century are ongoing, the body's reactions last longer than the few minutes needed to escape from a brief physical danger. Often, long-lasting stresses lead to chronic increases in blood pressure and blood glucose. This is due to the hypothalamus helping to "control" long-term stress by producing certain hormones. Unfortunately, the hypothalamus's actions can lead to long-term disorders such as hypertension, type 2 diabetes, stroke, heart disease, and kidney disease—disorders that can affect both your quality of life and your life span.

The system of *endocrine glands* includes the hypothalamus, pituitary, pineal, thyroid, parathyroid, thymus, adrenals, pancreas, ovaries (in women), and testes (in men). These glands secrete hormones, which are the body's chemical messengers. Circulated mostly through the bloodstream, hormones affect the function of every organ in the body, including your brain and gut. It is worth noting, however, that microbes produce chemicals that are similar to hormones in that they produce signals. These chemicals have an effect on the adrenal and pituitary glands, the hypothalamus, the thyroid, and the pineal glands. The hormones and chemicals produced by the glands and microbes all play a role in our growth and development, metabolism, reproduction, and moods. (For specific information on how the glands react in times of stress, see the inset on page 19.)

THE CONNECTION

As you've learned, the connection between the gut, the microbiome, and the brain depends on chemical messengers secreted by your glands. If you are experiencing stomach or intestinal distress, such as indigestion or acid reflux, a message is sent to the brain. Likewise, if the brain has a problem, such as depression or stress, it sends a message to the gut. In other words, what's happening in your gut affects your mental state, and your mental health affects your gut. Mental stress even affects your microbiome by causing gut issues that alter the kinds and numbers of bacteria in the GI tract.

WHEN THINGS GO WRONG

When your gut microbiome becomes overloaded with bad bacteria or depleted of healthy bacteria, as you might expect, intestinal problems like nausea and diarrhea may occur. Other bowel diseases, such as inflammatory bowel disease (IBD), Crohn's disease, and ulcerative colitis, may also develop.

As you learned on page 16, however, the body's bacteria affect a host of functions. Therefore, it should not be surprising that an imbalanced microbiome can impact the body far beyond the GI tract. For instance, your immune system, which enables you to fight disease, can be hampered by a poor microbiome. Your microbiome may also cause or exacerbate asthma, which is far more common (and lethal) in Blacks than Whites. New research also shows that altered microbes play a role in behavioral disorders such as autism, anxiety, and depression.

Exciting scientific research has also discovered a relationship between your gut microbes and chronic health problems such as obesity and type 2 diabetes. For instance, a decrease in the relative abundance of one species of gut bacteria, Bacteroides, is strikingly evident in obesity. And obesity, as you will learn in later chapters, is strongly associated with type 2 diabetes.

A poor microbiome can also promote heart disease. When people eat a standard Western diet—which is high in processed foods and low in beneficial fiber—the microbes metabolize certain dietary elements to create a toxic chemical associated with hardening of the arteries, also called *atherosclerosis*. In this condition, the substance plaque builds up in your blood vessels, increasing your blood pressure. If part of the plaque breaks off and travels to your heart, a heart attack occurs. Plaque that travels to the brain can result in a stroke. Both strokes and heart attacks—which can cause disability or early death—are all too common in Blacks.

Your microbiome can also contribute to autoimmune diseases, in which your immune system attacks your own healthy tissues, causing them to be damaged or destroyed. Some autoimmune diseases you may be familiar with are rheumatoid arthritis, which affects your joints; and multiple sclerosis (MS), in which chemicals attack the protective covering of the nerves, causing communication problems between the brain and the body. Lupus and celiac disease are also considered autoimmune disorders.

MAINTAINING THE RIGHT BALANCE IN YOUR GMB

Now you know how important it is to keep your microbiome happy and functioning normally. Fortunately, by modifying your diet to avoid the foods that destroy good bacteria and include the foods that allow healthy bacteria to thrive, you can do a great deal to maintain a beneficial microbiome.

Foods to Avoid

A number of foods should be avoided because of their adverse effects on the microbiome. Chief among these are highly processed foods such as white bread and white rice. Processed foods tend to lack the fiber that feeds good bacteria. Fried foods, which promote the growth of bad bacteria, should also be avoided. Similarly, it's important to steer clear of foods high in sugar and high-fructose corn syrup (such as soft drinks and many processed foods), as they decrease the numbers of good bacteria. While artificial sweeteners seem like a great way of avoiding sugar, they, too, have been shown to alter your microbiome. Finally, avoid trans and hydrogenated fats—common ingredients in processed foods—because they are known to destroy the good bacteria and increase the bad.

Foods to Eat

If you read the above discussion of foods to avoid, you know that processed foods—which are low in fiber—can damage your microbiome. It shouldn't be surprising, therefore, that the foods that help good bacteria to thrive—vegetables, beans and legumes, nuts, and fruits—are high in fiber. Why are high-fiber foods so helpful to the microbiome? Fiber is made up of long chains of carbohydrates that are difficult to digest, and thus end up intact in the lower intestine. There, the fiber is turned into short-chain fatty acids, which are used by your intestinal cells to make energy (food) for themselves and to contribute energy to other parts of the body. Dietary fiber that helps nourish the growth of good bacteria is known as *prebiotic fiber.*

Foods that lead to the production of short-chain fatty acids are also thought to play a key role in the prevention and treatment of *metabolic syndrome,* which is a group of disorders that include high blood pressure, elevated blood sugar, high cholesterol, and excess body weight around the waist. Metabolic syndrome is a precursor to diabetes and is strongly associated with heart disease and stroke, as well. Short-chain fatty acids also play a role in preventing bowel disorders and certain types of cancer.

Some foods actually provide live bacteria that can directly benefit your microbiome. These foods—which include sauerkraut, cheese, kimchi (spicy pickled cabbage), yogurt, and kefir—are known as *probiotic foods* because they actually contain live bacteria.

Probiotic Supplements

In addition to eating fiber-rich foods and foods containing live bacteria, you can support a healthy microbiome by taking *probiotic supplements*, which provide beneficial bacteria in the form of tablets, powders, or capsules. Many types of bacteria are used in probiotics. For the greatest benefit, you should choose a product that provides at least five different types of bacteria and more than 70 billion colonies. In my household, we take probiotics that have at least ten types of bacteria and over 100 billion colonies. Avoid "cheap" probiotics or supplements that contain only one type of bacteria. In the case of probiotics, more is better—more forms of bacteria and more colonies. The better supplements cost more, but aren't you worth it?

Although most people can benefit from probiotics, be aware that some people should avoid them. If you take immune suppression drugs, are undergoing treatment for a fungal infection, have a weak immune system, or have been diagnosed with pancreatitis, do not take probiotic supplements.

CONCLUSION

This chapter started out by comparing your Gut-Microbiome-Brain Connection to the workings of a car. When you don't give your car the right oil or gas, it will break down. If your battery is weak, your engine will have trouble starting. But if you give your car the fuel that it needs, it will run beautifully and serve you for many years.

So it is with your body. The fact is that for decades, Black people have suffered from disabling disorders and died too young because they were not aware of the steps they could take to improve their health. By simply knowing how your body works and giving it the fuel it needs to be at its best, you can free yourself from a number of health problems. Your GMB Connection was designed to keep you healthy. You have the responsibility to avoid gumming up the works.

The following chapters focus on the most common health problems found among members of our community. Although the problems are varied, the fact is that they are all connected through the issues discussed in this chapter. Most important, by making a few commonsense changes in your diet, you can avoid many of these problems and enjoy a healthier, happier life.

TIMELINES
FROM AFRICA TO
THE PRE-CIVIL WAR YEARS

1619 to 1730. Existing records of slave traders show mostly indifference to the well-being of their human cargo. The health of those Africans who had been brought to the American colonies and purchased as "property" was measured only by their ability to work and, in the case of enslaved women, their ability to reproduce. Medical problems and injuries were treated not out of compassion, but out of necessity, to preserve the slaves' value as property. And while we do not know what treatments were used to restore their health, the records that are available do reveal the brutal causes of their illnesses—"massive overwork, poor food, poor clothing, poor housing, inadequate sanitation, and overexposure to the elements."

1731 to 1860. By the 1700s, slavery was well entrenched in the nation's economy. Ironically, it was Crispus Attucks, a man of African descent who had escaped slavery, who was the first to lose his life on March 5, 1770 during the Boston Massacre. This was the first clash between the American colonists and the British Army and would pave the way for the American Revolution.

When America finally gained its independence, the years that followed saw the establishment of hospitals, medical schools, and the medical profession. Yet as the study of medicine progressed in this country, slaves were still considered property and viewed as less than human, without any right to receive the healthcare available at the time. Doctors had little interest in the treatment and healing of slaves. And as the first half of the 1800s moved forward, the cruelty to African slaves increased. Instead of being cared for as patients, Blacks were used for training purposes and experimentation.

For example, James Marion Sims (1813–1883), a Southern-born slaveholder, is credited as being the "father of modern gynecology." To earn that title, he performed surgical procedures on enslaved women without the use of anesthesia, because it was believed that Blacks did not feel pain and that their suffering was of no importance. He was not alone in his view of Blacks as inferior beings. It was an attitude that dominated the training of medical students as well as White society in general.

Both the *Baltimore Medical and Surgical Journal* and the *Western and Southern Medical Recorder* reported that between 1833 and 1858, several surgical experiments were performed on slaves in the study of treatments for injuries, birth defects, and tumors. These experiments were performed not to improve the well-being of the slaves but to use them as guinea pigs. In some cases, medical schools trafficked in slavery specifically to have subjects for use in their anatomy courses.

While there were doctors that served both Black freedmen and slaves, the vast majority of White healers did not. It would take decades to undo this inhuman treatment of the men and women of African descent.

2

Obesity

"Obesity isn't some simple, discrete issue. There's no one cause we can pinpoint. There's no one program we can fund to make it go away. Rather, it's an issue that touches on every aspect of how we live and how we work."
—Michelle Obama

There is no question that body image is important to our Black community—from our hairstyles to our clothing to our body language. How we choose to see ourselves greatly contributes to both our mental and physical well-being. However, we seem to have a blind spot when it comes to our body size. Growing up among family members and neighbors who may be overweight can provide a distorted view of what "normal" should look like.

Yes, Aunt Corinne had a beautiful face and was definitely a really "big" woman, but everyone loved her sense of humor, the way her body shook when she laughed, her kindness, and the meals she would prepare for us on holidays. Her dying at age fifty-five of a heart attack was definitely a surprise to everyone—but it should not have surprised us at all. That extra weight she had carried around since childhood was a ticking time bomb that cut her life short—as it has for millions of African Americans who are overweight.

The more you know about the dangers of any extra pounds you have on your body, the greater incentive you will have to do something about it. This is what this chapter is all about.

RECOGNIZING YOU HAVE A PROBLEM

Other people may tell us that we've gained a few pounds, but too many of us tend to laugh it off or ignore it completely. For some women, a big body may be a sign of sexiness. For some men, the extra weight may be a sign of success. It's easy to make excuses for extra pounds, but regardless of how you think you look or what you think your weight says about you, you need to pay attention to symptoms that may be telling you that something is very wrong. Consider just a few of the problems that are often associated with excess weight:

- Being unable to stand for a long period of time

- Constant knee and joint pain

- Feeling your heart race unexpectedly

- Shortness of breath when going up stairs

We will explore the problems associated with excess weight a little later in the chapter. Just as important, as you read this chapter, you will realize that while your behavior (and other factors) may have led to weight problems, you have the power to change—to become healthier, avoid the conditions associated with obesity, and extend your time on this planet.

HOW OVERWEIGHT ARE YOU?

Being overweight is defined as "weight that is higher than what is considered as a healthy weight for a given height." In the past, obesity was often defined as being 20 percent over ideal weight. This was based on your height, age, and gender. However, as technology progressed, so did the way medical researchers began to measure body weight.

Today, healthcare workers use the Body Mass Index, or BMI, to establish normal body weight. Under this numerical system, you are categorized as normal, overweight, obese, or extremely obese.

You may have seen this number on a printed sheet your doctor gave you, or your doctor may have discussed your BMI with you.

Establishing Your Body Mass Index (BMI)

By determining your BMI, you can see which of the categories just listed you fall into. Fortunately, this is simple with the use of Table 2.1 (see following page). In the left-hand column, locate your height in inches. Then move along that row to find your weight.

If you discover you are in the obese or extreme obesity category, you are not alone. In the United States, about 42 percent of adult Americans are obese, contributing to up to 365,000 obesity-related deaths every year. In addition, since 1980, the number of overweight children in this country has doubled, while the number of overweight adolescents has tripled. And in the Black community, the obesity numbers are even worse. African-American women have the highest rates of obesity compared with other racial groups in the United States, with four out of five Black women being obese. Statistics also show that Black children between the ages of six and seventeen are more likely to be overweight than their White peers.

As Black Americans, this health problem should be one of our top concerns. But instead of recognizing and dealing with the problem, we allow it to open the door to the deadly diseases that are killing so many of our men and women.

CAUSES OF OVERWEIGHT/OBESITY

If you are overweight, it would be easy to blame yourself, but that would be not only too simple but also wrong. In fact, there are many reasons—both personal and cultural—why this has happened. It is important to recognize how you have gotten to this point. The following nine factors may each have played their part.

FOOD ADVERTISING. Companies spend millions of dollars on ads that influence how we see "junk food" products, and these ads have a major impact on our behavior and buying habits. Unfortunately, many of the foods being promoted are highly addictive,

Table 2.1. Body Mass Index

	Normal						Overweight					Obese					
BMI	19	20	21	22	23	24	25	26	27	28	29	30	31	32	33	34	35
Height (inches)							Body Weight (pounds)										
58	91	96	100	105	110	115	119	124	129	134	138	143	148	153	158	162	167
59	94	99	104	109	114	119	124	128	133	138	143	148	153	158	163	168	173
60	97	102	107	112	118	123	128	133	138	143	148	153	158	163	168	174	179
61	100	106	111	116	122	127	132	137	143	148	153	158	164	169	174	180	185
62	104	109	115	120	126	131	136	142	147	153	158	164	169	175	180	186	191
63	107	113	118	124	130	135	141	146	152	158	163	169	175	180	186	191	197
64	110	116	122	128	134	140	145	151	157	163	169	174	180	186	192	197	204
65	114	120	126	132	138	144	150	156	162	168	174	180	186	192	198	204	210
66	118	124	130	136	142	148	155	161	167	173	179	186	192	198	204	210	216
67	121	127	134	140	146	153	159	166	172	178	185	191	198	204	211	217	223
68	125	131	138	144	151	158	164	171	177	184	190	197	203	210	216	223	230
69	128	135	142	149	155	162	169	176	182	189	196	203	209	216	223	230	236
70	132	139	146	153	160	167	174	181	188	195	202	209	216	222	229	236	243
71	136	143	150	157	165	172	179	186	193	200	208	215	222	229	236	243	250
72	140	147	154	162	169	177	184	191	199	206	213	221	228	235	242	250	258
73	144	151	159	166	174	182	189	197	204	212	219	227	235	242	250	257	265
74	148	155	163	171	179	186	194	202	210	218	225	233	241	249	256	264	272
75	152	160	168	176	184	192	200	208	216	224	232	240	248	256	264	272	279
76	156	164	172	180	189	197	205	213	221	230	238	246	254	263	271	279	287

36	37	38	39	40	41	42	43	44	45	46	47	48	49	50	51	52	53	54
				Extreme Obesity														
				Body Weight (pounds)														
172	177	181	186	191	196	201	205	210	215	220	224	229	234	239	244	248	253	258
178	183	188	193	198	203	208	212	217	222	227	232	237	242	247	252	257	262	267
184	189	194	199	204	209	215	220	225	230	235	240	245	250	255	261	266	271	276
190	195	201	206	211	217	222	227	232	238	243	248	254	259	264	269	275	280	285
196	202	207	213	218	224	229	235	240	246	251	256	262	267	273	278	284	289	295
203	208	214	220	225	231	237	242	248	254	259	265	270	278	282	287	293	299	304
209	215	221	227	232	238	244	250	256	262	267	273	279	285	291	296	302	308	314
216	222	228	234	240	246	252	258	264	270	276	282	288	294	300	306	312	318	324
223	229	235	241	247	253	260	266	272	278	284	291	297	303	309	315	322	328	334
230	236	242	249	255	261	268	274	280	287	293	299	306	312	319	325	331	338	344
236	243	249	256	262	269	276	282	289	295	302	308	315	322	328	335	341	348	354
243	250	257	263	270	277	284	291	297	304	311	318	324	331	338	345	351	358	365
250	257	264	271	278	285	292	299	306	313	320	327	334	341	348	355	362	369	376
257	265	272	279	286	293	301	308	315	322	329	338	343	351	358	365	372	379	386
265	272	279	287	294	302	309	316	324	331	338	346	353	361	368	375	383	390	397
272	280	288	295	302	310	318	325	333	340	348	355	363	371	378	386	393	401	408
280	287	295	303	311	319	326	334	342	350	358	365	373	381	389	396	404	412	420
287	295	303	311	319	327	335	343	351	359	367	375	383	391	399	407	415	423	431
295	304	312	320	328	336	344	353	361	369	377	385	394	402	410	418	426	435	443

meaning that they contain large amounts of salt and sugar, which our bodies learn to crave. By making us believe that these products represent the good times in our lives, ads train us to view these foods as necessary for our personal enjoyment. From cakes and cookies to chips and dips—from sodas and ice cream to oversized heroes—we fall for it, hook, line, and sinker. The result is bad eating habits and extra pounds.

FOOD DESERTS VERSUS FOOD OASES. Where you live and where you do your grocery shopping play an important role in what you eat. The term *food oases* refers to communities whose supermarkets provide large arrays of fresh foods, organic fruits and vegetables, and meats that have little or no antibiotics or hormones. But the US Department of Agriculture estimates that at least 23.5 million people in the United States live in *food desert* communities. If you live in a food desert, you are farther than one mile from a supermarket that offers a large variety of healthy foods.

National supermarket chains often decline to locate their retail operations in poorer communities. Instead, these areas are a draw for small grocery stores and fast food chains that do not have to compete against large supermarkets. They cater to minority communities by selling cheaper, lower-quality foods that often contain high levels of pesticides, herbicides, antibiotics, and hormones. They also sell lots of soda, beer, and cigarettes, all of which are big money makers. Of course, these are products that are killing the people who consume them. The bottom line is that poorer underserved communities have limited access to the high-quality, affordable, nutritious foods that promote wellness.

GENETICS. Research has proven that genetics plays a role in obesity, contributing to an individual's susceptibility to weight gain. This, of course, doesn't mean that the food you eat doesn't play a role. Eating too much food normally adds excess weight to your body. However, if your metabolism—which is directly related to your genes—burns off calories more quickly, you may avoid gaining weight even if you have a high-calorie diet. If, on the other hand, your metabolism is slow, the same diet is likely to put on excess pounds. The next time you are sitting around the dinner table at a family get-together, take a look around you. Are your family members all average weight or are they obese? If many of them are overweight, genetics may be a factor. This doesn't mean that you can't lose weight, but it may mean that you have to work harder to shed those excess pounds.

Research has shown that men descended from West Africa tend to be thin, while the women from the same area tend to be heavier around the middle, suggesting that gender may also play a role.

HYPOTHYROIDISM. Located in the neck, the thyroid gland is responsible for producing hormones that regulate the body's metabolism. *Hypothyroidism*, or an underactive thyroid gland, can cause weight gain as well as fatigue, dry skin, and poor memory. Since the symptoms are seemingly unrelated, hypothyroidism often goes undiagnosed for years. If you suspect that you may be suffering from this illness or have a family history of hypothyroidism, discuss it with your doctor, who can test your thyroid function. This problem can be effectively treated with inexpensive medication.

MEDICATIONS. Certain drugs can cause weight gain. They do this in a number of ways—by increasing hunger, water retention, and fat storage; by lowering metabolism; and/or by causing fatigue, which can decrease your daily activity. Drugs that can have this effect include anti-inflammatories, antidepressants, high blood pressure pills, pills for diabetes, and seizure medications. Ask your doctor or pharmacist if the medications you are taking can lead to weight gain.

LACK OF SLEEP. Sleep is critical to virtually every aspect of health and wellness. During sleep, the brain tries to put your body back in order by neutralizing toxins and cleaning up and disposing of wastes from the day's work. Sleep promotes physical health and recovery, with direct effects on almost all systems of the body. Sleep also affects cognitive function, attention, and memory and plays an integral role in emotional health.

Researchers have found that Blacks sleep fewer hours than Whites. Sometimes, a vicious cycle is involved, in which less sleep causes increased stress, which in turn leads to insomnia. Reduced sleep can also be the result of neighborhood noise or of worry-inducing financial concerns. Blacks are also more likely to be shift-workers, which interferes with regular bedtime hours and sleep rhythms.

Sleep and weight are strongly associated, with short sleep times increasing the likelihood of being overweight by 16 percent and increasing obesity by 32 percent. This alone may motivate you to take steps to improve your sleep.

YOUR MICROBIOME. In Chapter 1, you learned the importance of your microbiome—the microbes (mostly bacteria) that live in your gut. Chapter 1 also explained that diet can play an important role in keeping your microbiome healthy, which, in turn, will keep you healthy. Conversely, a poor diet can have an adverse effect on your microbiome, and thus adversely affect your health. What does this have to do with obesity? It has been found that a high-fat diet actually alters the microbiome by increasing certain families of bacteria (Firmicutes and Proteobacteria) and lowering levels of another family of bacteria (Bacteroidetes). This, in turn, promotes weight gain.

Fortunately, there's a great deal you can do to keep your microbiome populated by beneficial bacteria that support a healthy weight. One epidemiological study, for instance, showed that eating yogurt, which is rich in "good" bacteria, helped prevent age-associated weight gain. So by following the guidelines for improving gut health that begin on page 21, you will not only promote better health in general but also make it easier to shed unwanted pounds.

STRESS. Obesity is a complex condition caused by multiple factors, which, not surprisingly, include emotional stress. As you may know from your own experience, many people eat more than usual when they are bored, angry, or upset. While stress is common throughout society, the following can cause African Americans to experience more than the usual stress:

- Cultural eating of calorie-rich foods

- Discrimination in obtaining affordable housing

- Food deserts and poor-quality foods

- Income inequities

- Lack of free time to exercise

- Living in toxic communities

- Minimal access to childcare

- Poor access to healthcare

- Poor access to quality education

- Stressful jobs

Once you understand that all these factors can contribute to stress and, in turn, to weight gain, you can start making the changes you need to get your weight under control.

CULTURAL CAUSES. Unfortunately, this one is on us. Any one of the issues already discussed can contribute to weight gain, but one of the biggest problems in the Black community today is the acceptance of overweight and obesity as the norm. Within the African-American community, curvy, overweight women are often considered more appealing than average- or under-weight women. There is almost a reverse distortion of body image, with overweight women fighting weight loss and slender women wanting to gain weight in order to be considered more attractive. Over time, this preference can be changed by understanding that a leaner body means a healthier body.

Sometimes a group's cultural cuisine can negatively affect its health, and this is certainly the case in the African-American community. The fatty, salty, and simply unhealthy cooking methods that characterize "soul food" are proving to be a giant stumbling block for African Americans who want to lose weight. But you need not abandon your traditions to improve your well-being. The same foods that have been giving you comfort over the years can be prepared in a healthier manner. Instead of deep-frying your vegetables, roast them in the oven or sauté them in a low-sodium broth. Instead of using bacon grease and butter in your cooking, substitute olive or canola oil. Just as important, taste your food before you add salt or butter for flavor. Over time, by using less salt and fat, you will find your tastes changing. Small adjustments to your favorite meals can make a world of difference to your waistline and your general health.

THE EFFECTS OF OBESITY

Whether you find extra weight attractive or unattractive, the unfortunate fact is that excess pounds—especially when they reach the level of obesity—can (and often do) lead to a wide range of serious health problems. According to the Centers for Disease Control (CDC), the following all-too-common disorders are directly caused by or related to obesity:

- Body pain
- Coronary heart disease
- Depression, anxiety, and other mental disorders
- Gallbladder disease
- High blood pressure (hypertension)
- High LDL (bad) cholesterol, low HDL (good) cholesterol, or high levels of triglycerides
- Osteoarthritis (a breakdown of cartilage and bone within a joint)
- Sleep apnea and breathing problems
- Stroke
- Type 2 diabetes
- Various forms of cancer

Whether you are Black or White, being diagnosed with any of these health disorders is life-altering. If you are African-American, however, these disorders are all too common and kill a disproportionate number of people in your community. If this isn't enough cause for concern, there are two more issues that must be discussed—the effects of obesity on your hormones, and the effects of obesity on infant health and mortality.

Effects of Obesity on Hormones

As you learned in Chapter 1, the endocrine glands produce hormones that go directly into the bloodstream and act as chemical messengers. Fat cells can also secrete a group of hormones, called *adipocytokines*, which affect glucose and fat metabolism, reproduction, and cardiovascular function. Some of these hormones affect your weight. For example, leptin, a hormone secreted by fat cells, communicates with the brain to control your appetite. However, if you are overweight or obese, this communication is altered. The leptin no longer signals your brain to feel full, so instead of decreasing your food intake, you keep eating.

Another hormone, *adiponectin*, is also affected by obesity. Normally, adiponectin increases insulin sensitivity so that the body responds properly to blood sugar levels. In the case of obesity, however, lower amounts of adiponectin are produced, making the cells more resistant to insulin. This increases blood sugar levels and, over time, can lead to diabetes. Your fat metabolism—that is, the amount of fat you burn up—is also affected, leading to more plaque buildup in your arteries. This sets the stage for high blood pressure (hypertension) and perhaps a heart attack or stroke. Overweight/obesity can even affect the system that regulates fluids in your body, which can also lead to hypertension.

Some effects of obesity on hormones are specific to women, whose menstrual cycles can be altered. Periods can stop, or there may be an increase in flow and/or an increase or decrease in cycle frequency. There may also be an increase in facial hair growth. Alterations of hormones may also occur in men, but they are less obvious; nevertheless, the effects are there.

Effects of Obesity on Maternal and Infant Health

If all that was discussed above isn't bad enough, tragically, maternal obesity can lead to problems during pregnancy and increased health problems for babies. In mothers, a high BMI increases the risk of miscarriage and stillbirth, gestational diabetes, high blood pressure, cardiac dysfunction, sleep apnea, and the need for a C-section. In babies, maternal obesity increases the risk of birth defects, being significantly larger than average (fetal macrosomia), impaired growth, childhood asthma, and childhood obesity.

Another problem for overweight/obese women who become pregnant is that toxic chemicals from their food, air, and water that enter their bloodstream are stored in fat cells. There, they accumulate and are transported through the placenta to their fetus. These toxic chemicals are known to cause fetal and pregnancy abnormalities.

A group of scientists tested cord blood from ten babies of color for toxic chemicals. Every sample was contaminated and revealed 232 different industrial compounds. These chemicals are known to cause infertility, miscarriages, obesity, diabetes, and even genetic alterations that will be passed on to the baby's children, grandchildren, and even great grandchildren. Chapter 10 is devoted to toxic chemicals that affect Blacks more than Whites because of their contaminated neighborhoods, food, and water.

HOW TO LOSE WEIGHT

If you are overweight, your doctor may have told you, "You must lose some weight now! Your life is at stake!" Your doc may have given you a specific diet to follow or suggested that you join a weight-loss program. While changing your diet is an important part of any weight-loss program, there many additional things you can do to drop unwanted pounds and, along the way, improve your overall health. The discussion below begins by highlighting two diets that have been shown to work. It then looks at other ways in which you can help your body reach and maintain a healthy weight. You can do this!

Changing Your Diet

If you have decided that a weight-loss diet will help you reach your goals, I recommend either the American Heart Association Diet or the Mediterranean Diet, which I describe much more fully in Chapter 9. (See page 166.) These two diets have been used successfully to improve the well-being of millions of people in both Europe and the United States. Both plans guide you to healthier meals composed of fresh fruits and vegetables, whole grains, lean meat, milk and cheese, unprocessed nuts, and legumes.

Ask your doctor if he or she has handouts that provide information about these diets. You can also find information on these diets as well as support on the Internet. There, you'll find what is allowed, what is not allowed, recipes, guidelines for grocery shopping, and more. (For some of the best websites on these diets, see page 285 of the Resources.)

Choosing the Right Foods and Avoiding the Wrong Ones

Whether you choose to stick to a prescribed diet or count calories, it's important to choose the right foods and avoid the wrong ones. I suggest that my patients avoid processed foods such as fast foods, sugary beverages and other sugar-laden foods, packaged snack foods, white bread, desserts, and high-fat foods. Decreasing your sugar intake will help you avoid diabetes and obesity. If you have hypertension you will need to lower your salt intake. You will also need to stop using your salt shaker at the table and to drastically reduce the salt you add in the kitchen. We will be covering more about nutrition in Chapter 9.

Making Exercise Part of Your Life

As you learned earlier in this chapter, excess body fat influences the hormones that regulate appetite. Thus, an obese person's hunger may not be satisfied quite as easily as the hunger of a slimmer person. In other words, weight begets weight. But you also learned that active people burn more calories than people who are more sedentary. So it's easy to understand that to reach a healthier weight, you must get off the couch and start moving! Your life may actually depend on it.

Exercise will decrease your appetite and burn calories. Your breathing and endurance will improve, and you will start to feel better. You want to increase your heart rate during exercise, but if all you are able to do is to go for a short walk at the beginning, that's fine. Exercising may be easier if you start after you have lost five to seven pounds. If the weather is bad, you can walk indoors and up and down stairs, or you can walk in your local mall. As your strength and endurance improves, increase the length of your walk and your speed. You can even add arm movements to

COUNTING CALORIES TO LOSE WEIGHT

Instead of following a specific diet, such as the Mediterranean Diet discussed on page 169, some people prefer to budget their calories. A calorie is a unit of energy. To gain weight, you need to eat more calories than you currently eat, and to lose weight, you need to eat fewer calories. Your calorie needs depend on your age, sex, and physical activity. Generally, men need more than women, younger people need more than older, and more active people need more calories than less active people because physical activity burns calories. (For a general guide to calories needed per day to maintain current weight, see Table 2.2.) The bottom line is that if you cut about 500 to 1,000 calories a day from your current diet, you would lose about one to two pounds per week.

To learn how many calories are in a particular packaged food— such as beans, soup, crackers, etc.—look at the Nutrition Facts label on the package. There, you'll find the number of calories in a serving, as well as the amount of fat, sodium, carbohydrates, protein, and sometimes other nutrients. Be sure to pay attention to the serving size, which may be smaller than the amount you're actually eating. If you find that you are eating two servings, for instance, you will be taking in twice the calories provided by a single serving.

increase your heart rate. To make exercise more enjoyable, ask a friend—or several friends—to join you.

While walking is a great way to increase physical activity, of course, it's not the only way. If you like to dance, choose some music that will get you moving, and have fun. Another good option is to join a gym or your local YMCA.

Experts recommend that you engage in moderate aerobic activity for 20 to 30 minutes a day; or, if you're engaging in vigorous aerobic activity, you exercise for a little more than 10 minutes a day. (See the inset on page 42.) You can also combine moderate and vigorous activity. Remember to gradually build up your time and

Table 2.2. Calorie Needs per Day by Age, Sex, and Physical Activity						
	MALES			FEMALES		
Age in Years	Sedentary	Moderately Active	Active	Sedentary	Moderately Active	Active
30	2,400	2,600	3,000	1,800	2,000	2,400
40	2,400	2,600	2,800	1,800	2,000	2,200
50	2,200	2,400	2,800	1,800	2,000	2,200
60	2,200	2,400	2,800	1,600	1,800	2,200
70	2,000	2,200	2,600	1,600	1,800	2,200
76+	2,000	2,200	2,400	1,600	1,800	2,000

From Appendix 2 Estimated Calorie Needs, Dietary Guidelines, 2020.

Of course, calorie counting works only if you record the amount of calories consumed throughout the day. To help you keep track of your calories, try one of these free apps: MyFitness-Pal, Loselt!, FatSecret, Cronometer, and SparkPeople.

UNDERSTANDING THE DIFFERENT
EXERCISE INTENSITIES

The section on exercise that begins on page 39 may use a handful of terms with which you are not familiar. Let's look at those terms.

Aerobic activity (meaning "with oxygen") is exercise that increases cardiac fitness by increasing your breathing and heart rate. Brisk walking, cycling, swimming, and running are all aerobic activities.

Moderate exercise feels somewhat hard. Your breathing increases, but you are not out of breath. After about 10 minutes, you develop a mild sweat. You can talk with a friend during this activity, but you can't sing!

Vigorous or heavy exercise feels harder. Your breathing is deep and fast. You develop a sweat after a few minutes. During this type of exercise, you can't say more than a few words without stopping to breathe.

intensity. When you're comfortable doing vigorous exercise, you may want to add strength training.

If you are overweight or obese; if you have any kind of chronic health condition; or if you simply haven't exercised in years, be sure to check with your healthcare provider before you start to exercise. Keep in mind that you will find even moderate activity difficult at first. However, making exercise a part of your weekly routine will lift your spirits by releasing endorphins, the feel-good hormones.

Drinking More Water

Water is an often overlooked tool in the fight against obesity. By increasing your water intake by about 16 ounces per day, you will boost your metabolic rate by 30 percent. The consumption of eight 8-ounce glasses of water per day burns about 70 calories, while dehydration slows down fat metabolism. Water is also required to flush out the toxins released from your body by weight loss.

Finally, drinking water with a meal helps you lose weight by making you feel full sooner, which causes you to eat less.

Most experts recommend eight 8-ounce glasses of water per day. You may feel the need to drink a few glasses more, though, depending on your weight and your level of physical activity.

Getting More Sleep

Studies conducted at the New York University School of Medicine have revealed that a lack of sleep can have a profound effect on hormones. Sleep disturbances can significantly decrease levels of the appetite-suppressant leptin and raise levels of the appetite-stimulant ghrelin. Studies have also shown a connection between sleep deprivation and an elevated consumption of calorie-dense foods. Fortunately, just as sleep deprivation can contribute to weight gain, the treatment of sleep disorders contributes to both weight loss and increased energy. To benefit from sleep, try to get seven to eight hours of rest per night.

Summoning Your Willpower

Underlying any suggestion I have made is the need to stick with the weight-loss tactics you choose. When we face racism in our daily lives, I understand how stressful, frustrating, and hurtful that can be. We may want to scream or strike out, but for most of us, we find it within ourselves to move on. That is not weakness. That's our willpower at work. We make our goal of moving ahead in our lives a priority. We resist the urge to lose our cool, because we are better than that. We recognize racism as pure ignorance.

In exactly the same way, you have it within yourself to resist the urge to eat foods that you know are bad for you. Why? Because Black lives matter, starting with your life and those of the people you love.

Taking Helpful Supplements

Supplements contain one or more ingredients—such as vitamins, minerals, herbs, or amino acids—that are not considered food and are intended to supplement your diet. They can be taken for a number of reasons, such as addressing a deficiency or helping to treat a specific condition. The supplements listed below have been found to support weight loss by affecting the production or metabolism of fat, boosting energy, and/or performing other important functions. For guidance in choosing the best-quality supplements and using them effectively, see the supplements guide on page 258.

Glisodin

Derived from cantaloupe extract and a wheat protein, glisodin helps you reduce fat production and neutralize the free radicals produced by your liver. (For more about free radicals, see the inset on page 47.) This supplement also increases energy production and reduces fatigue. I recommend taking 150 mg once or twice a day, depending on your particular need.

Glutathione

Some refer to glutathione (GSH) as your liver's best friend, but it is found in every cell in the body. Glutathione chemically neutralizes free radicals generated by obesity and exercise to help you safely reduce your weight. It also helps regenerate other antioxidants that neutralize free radicals, and it transports mercury and other toxic metals out of cells and the brain so that they can be excreted. Finally, glutathione regulates cell growth and cell death.

Foods naturally rich in glutathione are spinach, avocados, asparagus, and okra. The problem is that when these natural sources are processed during digestion, most of the glutathione is destroyed by stomach acids. Often, people aren't able to eat enough foods to make up for the glutathione deficiency. This is why I recommend a dose of 500 mg or 1,000 mg of glutathione per day. You can also increase your glutathione intake is by using the supplement N-Acetyl Cysteine (NAC), which is discussed on page 46.

Green Tea Extract

Green tea extract is known to support weight loss by improving metabolism and increasing the burning of fat, especially when paired with exercise. This ability is most likely a result of the combination

ABOUT WEIGHT-LOSS DRUGS

Right now, you may be thinking, "Why can't I just take a pill—a weight-loss drug? That would be so much easier than changing my diet!" I believe that weight-loss medications are dangerous, and I do not recommend them. Additionally, these drugs work only while you are taking them and do not solve the primary causes of overweight or obesity.

The most common diet pill is phentermine, which is part of the amphetamine (stimulant) family of drugs. Several years ago, phentermine was one of two drugs that were combined to form the anti-obesity medication fen-phen. This drug resulted in several deaths caused by primary high blood pressure in the lungs and heart valve problems. It has since been removed from the market. It has been suggested that phentermine alone can cause the same problems and harmful side effects. Considering all these facts, drugs, in my opinion, are not the answer to the problem of obesity.

of green tea's natural caffeine and the tea's other nutrients, especially the catechins—the most biologically active compounds in green tea. Green tea also provides benefits for people with type 2 diabetes. (See page 88 for more about green tea and diabetes.) I recommend adding 6 to 9 drops of green tea extract to 32 ounces of water and drinking the mixture throughout the day.

Greens Powder

A concentrated powder made of nutrient-dense green foods such as wheatgrass, kale, chlorella, and spirulina, greens powder is packed with healthful compounds called phytonutrients. During weight loss, greens not only provide nutrition but also alkalize your body, reducing the absorption of toxins and increasing the elimination of waste from your gastrointestinal tract. Read the manufacturer's instructions for dosage guidelines.

5-Hydroxytryptophan

Also known as 5-HTP, this amino acid is involved in the conversion of tryptophan to serotonin, a neurotransmitter responsible for mood regulation. Moreover, 5-HTP reduces your appetite, may reduce binge-eating, and promotes weight loss. It is also used to treat depression, anxiety, and sleep problems.

You can enjoy the benefits of 5-HTP by taking 50 mg two to three times a day. However, this supplement is not recommended if you are already taking other medications that increase serotonin levels, such certain antidepressants. If you are currently taking antidepressants and you nevertheless want to try 5-HTP, be sure to consult with your healthcare provider.

Irvingia Gabonensis

Fruit from the native West African irvingia gabonensis tree is similar to a mango and is used for food. The fiber-rich seeds, used to make supplements, are believed to help in weight loss by reducing cholesterol and glucose levels. Benefits of this supplement can be enjoyed by taking doses of 150 mg twice daily.

L-Theanine

As you know, when you are stressed, you often overeat. L-theanine is an amino acid that assists in managing anxiety and helps blunt the effects of the hormone cortisol, which increases when you are chronically stressed. This supplement has been found to promote relaxation without causing drowsiness. I recommend taking 100 mg of L-theanine three times a day.

N-Acetyl Cysteine (NAC)

Derived from the amino acid L-cysteine, N-acetyl cysteine (NAC) is effective at raising levels of the antioxidant glutathione, which neutralizes free radicals. (See page 47.) For most people, 1,000 mg a day of NAC substantially increases glutathione. For the rare patient who reacts to NAC, SAMe can be used.

FREE RADICALS AND ANTIOXIDANTS

As you'll learn when you read about the supplements that support weight loss, some supplements benefit you by fighting free radicals. Why is this important? Free radicals are unstable molecules that are normally produced in the body when the cells use oxygen to generate energy. These molecules can also form when toxic chemicals such as those in tobacco smoke or polluted air enter the body. While they are often "natural," and they do perform useful functions when present at low levels, at high levels, free radicals can damage cells and promote aging and related health problems, such as heart disease and cancer. Obesity itself is associated with an excessive number of free radicals, and exercise, which speeds up metabolism, generates even more free radicals.

Fortunately, supplements that provide substances known as antioxidants are able to neutralize free radicals so that they don't harm you. You can also benefit from antioxidants by eating fruits and vegetables, which contain these substances in the form of vitamins A, C, and E, and as phytochemicals (plant chemicals). By taking antioxidant-rich supplements, loading up on fruits and vegetables, and avoiding toxic chemicals such as those in tobacco, you can protect your body against the damaging effects of free radicals.

Reds Powder

Eating berries is known to help you lose weight, but if you can't eat these fruits, you can take reds powder. Made largely from powdered fruit, reds powder provides similar detoxifying properties as greens powder, along with the antioxidant protection of colorful foods such as raspberries, blueberries, cranberries, and pomegranates. Read the manufacturer's instructions for dosage guidelines.

Saffron

A spiced derived from the Crocus Sativus flower, saffron combats the emotional aspect of overeating by increasing serotonin levels in your body. Serotonin promotes a feeling of fullness while also alleviating stress and the onset of depression, all of which contribute to compulsive eating. Research has found that 30 mg of saffron taken twice daily can have a positive effect on weight loss.

Vitamin D

We all have vitamin D receptor cells throughout our body. These cells convert cholesterol into vitamin D once our skin is exposed to ultraviolet light from the sun. White people obtain only 10 percent of vitamin D from food, and the rest is made by their bodies. Nevertheless, many Whites need vitamin D supplementation. Because the pigmentation of Blacks reduces vitamin D production, deficiency is even more prevalent among African Americans.

The body produces two types of vitamin D, vitamin D_2 and D_3. Vitamin D_3 is the superior form because it is more easily absorbed and used by the cells of the body. There are three ways in which you can obtain D_3: from the body, which is a problem for most African Americans; from foods such as fortified milk and fatty fish; and from supplements.

Besides the well-established role of vitamin D to build strong bones and teeth, vitamin D_3 helps in the alleviation of diseases such as type 2 diabetes, kidney disease, and heart disease. Vitamin D_3 may also be useful in weight loss. In one study, insufficient vitamin D_3 was associated with stunted growth and increased weight in young girls. In another study, low levels of vitamin D_3 were linked to elevated weight, increased BMI, and a greater occurrence of type 2 diabetes. This research reflects the growing evidence of a strong relationship between low levels of vitamin D_3 and excess weight. Furthermore, this relationship seems to begin at an early age.

Vitamin D_3 supplements are relatively cheap. For most people, 2,000 IU to 5,000 IU per day of vitamin D_3 is beneficial. You can also ask your healthcare provider to test your vitamin D levels and prescribe a dosage based on your test results. Make sure that your physician orders the 25-OH vitamin D test, as this will give you the best indication of your vitamin D body stores.

CONCLUSION

Underlying almost all the problems we will discuss in the chapters that follow is the problem of obesity. In this chapter, you have already read about the many adverse effects that excess weight can have on your body. As frightening as this may be, you've also learned that there are many things you can do to shed pounds, from changing your diet to getting more sleep to reducing your stress. Something as simple as taking a walk each day can have a major positive effect over time.

I know that breaking life-long habits, such as the habit of eating the wrong foods, is never easy for anyone. It will be a struggle to reach a healthier weight, but you understand the meaning of struggle. Most people in the Black community have struggled against segregation, struggled to have our voices heard, and struggled to be given an equal playing field. The fight against excess weight is a very personal struggle that you can win. And I promise that it will pay off in so many ways.

TIMELINES
THE NIGHT DOCTORS

1865 to 1930. "Night Doctors" is the term given to the supposed kidnappers of Blacks for the purpose of dissection and experimentation in medical schools. According to some sources, the stories of the Night Doctors were folktales told to slaves by Southern slave owners to keep them from running off or to freedmen to keep them from moving to the North.

Before the Civil War, the use of slaves' bodies for dissection in medical schools was common. Slaves who died were likely to be buried in shallow graves located in potter's fields. It was easy for grave robbers to remove these bodies and sell them to the highest bidders. In Massachusetts, North Carolina, and Mississippi, laws were passed allowing for unclaimed bodies to be used by medical schools. The persistent attitudes towards Blacks as less than human, the need for bodies to be experimented on or dissected, and the money paid for these bodies were perfect incentives for grave robbers to procure bodies in any way they could.

After the Civil War, the possibility that things would dramatically change was highly unlikely, especially in the South. Beginning in the 1870s, branches of the Ku Klux Klan extended into nearly every Southern state to suppress the rights of Blacks through intimidation and violence. It was all too common for Blacks to disappear at night or to be found hanging from trees. So while the stories of the Night Doctors may have been fabricated to frighten Blacks, the history behind these tales was all too real.

3

Hypertension

*"There is no greater agony than bearing
an untold story inside you."*
—MAYA ANGELOU

Hypertension, commonly known as high blood pressure, has been called the "silent killer," and for good reason. This disease has no obvious symptoms to indicate that something is wrong. You may look and feel fine, but over time, hypertension can lead to heart attacks, strokes, kidney failure, and death. And while it affects over 75 million people in the United States, statistics show that African Americans are at the highest risk. Here are some of the facts about hypertension (HTN) that you need to know:

- Although African-American adults are 40-percent more likely to have high blood pressure, they are less likely than their non-Hispanic white counterparts to have their blood pressure under control.

- In 2017, African Americans were 20-percent more likely to die from heart disease than non-Hispanic whites.

- African-American women are 60 percent more likely to have high blood pressure than non-Hispanic white women.

This chapter will provide you with a better understanding of hypertension, the factors that contribute to its development, and the ways in which you can reduce your risk of this disorder. In

WHAT DO BLOOD PRESSURE READINGS MEAN?

Blood pressure (BP) is expressed as a combination of two numbers—120/80, for example. The first number—120, in this case—refers to the systolic pressure. *Systolic pressure* measures the force exerted by the blood on artery walls when the heart beats. The second number—80—refers to the diastolic pressure. *Diastolic pressure* measures the force exerted by the blood on artery walls while the heart is momentarily at rest between heartbeats. When the numbers are high, such as 150/120, this means that the heart needs to work much harder to push the blood through the body's network of arteries, veins, and capillaries. The table below shows you the range of blood pressure readings to help you determine where you stand.

Table 3.1. Blood Pressure Categories and Readings

Category	Systolic Pressure (first number)		Diastolic Pressure (second number)
Normal	Less than 120	and	Less than 80
Elevated	120–129	and	Less than 80
Stage 1 Hypertension	130–139	or	80–99
Stage 2 Hypertension	140 or higher	or	90 or higher
Hypertensive Crisis	Higher than 180	and/or	Higher than 120

If your doctor has asked you to check your blood pressure at home, make sure to write your numbers down so that you can track them and see the effect of the steps you're taking to control your BP. (See the inset on page 60 to learn more about monitoring BP.) Once you see your BP begin to decrease, it will encourage you to continue with your hypertension-lowering regimen.

avoiding or better managing hypertension, you will be taking a vitally important step towards preventing killer diseases such as heart attack and kidney failure, which too frequently follow a diagnosis of hypertension.

WHAT IS HYPERTENSION?

Hypertension is a condition of the cardiovascular system, which is responsible for carrying blood to every part of the body. The cardiovascular system is made up of the heart and blood vessels. The heart is basically a pump that pushes the blood in your body. Blood leaves the heart through vessels called *arteries*, is carried to and from tissues through vessels called *capillaries*, and returns to the heart through vessels called *veins*. As blood gets pumped into the arteries, it exerts pressure on the walls of those blood vessels. This force is appropriately called *blood pressure (BP)*. When our blood pressure readings are normal, this tells us that our hearts are pushing out blood with just the right force. However, when it takes more force for the heart to push the blood through the body, that additional pressure creates the condition referred to as high blood pressure. (See the inset on page 52 to learn about blood pressure readings.)

There are two types of hypertension: primary (essential) hypertension and secondary hypertension. *Primary hypertension* usually develops gradually over many years and is caused by a number of genetic and environmenal factors, including age, gender, race, family history, stress, excessive sodium or alcohol intake, poor diet, lack of exercise, and obesity. *Secondary hypertension* is usually caused by an underlying health condition such as kidney disease or a congenital heart disorder; or by the use of drugs, including birth control pills, cold and flu remedies, decongestants, and pain medications, as well as illegal drugs such as amphetamines and cocaine.

While hypertension is undoubtedly a problem for individuals of every color and ethnicity, it has become a signature condition of the Black community over the last few decades, occurring three to five times as often in Black Americans than it does in White Americans. As a result, there are much higher rates of stroke, kidney failure, and congestive heart failure—diseases that can occur as result of long-term hypertension—in the Black population than in the white population.

Even worse, doctors are now starting to see high blood pressure not only in Black adults, but also in Black adolescents. Because many healthcare providers still do not recognize the possibility of such an early onset of hypertension, they do not test for it. Ask your healthcare provider to measure your children's and teens' blood pressure routinely. The earlier this condition is diagnosed, the more likely it is that steps can be taken to control or eliminate it and avoid the health problems that it can cause.

HOW DOES THE BODY MAINTAIN THE RIGHT BLOOD PRESSURE?

The blood that flows through our arteries and veins delivers nutrition, oxygen, water, and hormones to every cell in our body. It also picks up and removes nitrogen and waste products so that they can be eliminated from the body. This is what keeps us alive. How does our body know how much pressure is needed to keep this flow moving at the right speed? When you think about it, it is a miracle of nature.

In blood vessels near the heart, sensors called *baroreceptors* provide the brain with information about blood volume and pressure. These sensors send signals to the heart, veins, and kidneys that make them increase or lower blood flow. Based on the signals, our blood vessels can expand or contract. When they expand, they provide more room for the blood to flow, lowering our blood pressure. When they contract, there is less space for the blood to flow, raising our blood pressure. To make sure that our blood can continue doing its job of providing our body with what it needs or removing what it doesn't, the heart either slows down or speeds up.

Our two kidneys also play an important role in blood pressure control. When blood pressure is increased, the kidneys remove more urine (essentially water) from the blood, which lowers our blood pressure by reducing the volume of blood that flows through the blood vessels. When there is a decrease in blood pressure, the kidneys remove less urine, thereby increasing blood pressure by increasing blood volume. The kidneys constantly make adjustments to keep our blood pressure at a normal level.

Our body's ability to coordinate this complex process is based on each person's biochemistry. What you want to remember is that the body is always striving to stay in balance, and we should avoid doing things that prevent it from doing its job.

WHAT CAUSES HYPERTENSION?

While no clear-cut cause of high blood pressure has been determined, research has identified a handful of factors that contribute to the problem. These issues include genetic predisposition; exposure to certain risk factors in the womb; vitamin D_3 deficiency; type 2 diabetes; atherosclerosis; lifestyle considerations such as lack of exercise, smoking, and stress; and the use of certain medications.

Genetic Predisposition

The Renin-Angiotensin-Aldosterone System (RAAS) is a hormone system that regulates blood pressure and fluid balance. Because of a genetic variant found in many people of African descent, when they consume too much salt, it inappropriately stimulates their RAAS to cause excess sodium (salt) retention and higher levels of fluid in the circulatory system. This creates a fluid overload that increases blood pressure. Along with other factors, such as poor nutrition and excessive body weight, this genetic predisposition can take its toll over time. (To learn about the relationship of sodium to hypertension, see the inset on page 56.)

Prenatal Exposure to Lifestyle and Environmental Risks

As you've just read, the genes that individuals inherit from their ancestors play an important role in determining their blood pressure as adults. In addition, as a fetus develops in its mother's womb, it is exposed to a wide range of factors that can further increase

What's the Relationship Between Salt and High Blood Pressure?

When your bloodstream contains excess sodium (salt), it pulls water into your blood vessels, increasing your blood pressure. Some people—including about 75 percent of Black people—are especially sensitive to salt, which means that salt intake is likely to cause a dramatic rise in their blood pressure. (In contrast, people who are salt-resistant have little response to increased salt intake.) Age, weight, gender, and medical conditions like diabetes can also affect salt sensitivity. If you have high blood pressure, do your best to decrease your dietary salt, and speak to your doctor about taking a diuretic, which causes more water and sodium to be expelled from the body.

the odds of developing hypertension. For example, a recent study showed that if the pregnant mother is obese, is physically inactive, has a poor diet, drinks alcohol, or smokes cigarettes, her baby is at higher risk for eventually developing hypertension. In other words, the mother's lifestyle choices at the time of her pregnancy can affect the baby's future health.

In another study, it was shown that pregnant mothers who are exposed to environmental toxins also give birth to babies who are at higher risks of developing hypertension. The researchers concluded that there is a connection between high blood pressure and exposure of the fetus to environmental chemicals that include mercury, arsenic, lead, plastics, pesticides, persistent organic pollutants, and other toxins.

This information makes it's easier to understand why some African Americans are developing hypertension during childhood. When children are examined during a doctor's appointment, most physicians don't check the child's blood pressure. Maybe it's time we ask the doctor to do just that. Consider this: In most cases, children with hypertension will grow up exposed to air pollution—such as automobile exhaust, nitrogen dioxide, and small particles—that will make their condition even worse. That's why it's so important to diagnose this disorder early and take steps to combat it.

Vitamin D₃ Deficiency

Some studies suggest that a vitamin D_3 deficiency may lead to abnormally high levels of renin—one of the RAAS hormones that can cause hypertension. According to a report in *The Journal of Hypertension*, at least 50 percent of all cases of hypertension in dark-skinned Americans can be linked to low levels of vitamin D_3.

Sedentary Lifestyle

Research shows that a sedentary lifestyle contributes to an elevation in blood pressure. A study of 13,748 people revealed an increase in inflammation—which is associated with high blood pressure—in those who did not exercise, and a decrease in inflammation in those who did. In addition, patients who have had or are at risk of having a heart attack invariably show great improvements once they adopt a regular exercise regimen. Simply put, exercise is known to reduce blood pressure in people with hypertension as well as in those who have normal blood pressure. Exercise not only brings down your blood pressure but also improves other health problems, including obesity and insulin resistance, which are themselves contributors to hypertension.

Smoking

Although most people associate smoking with lung cancer, this nasty habit also substantially increases your risk of developing high blood pressure. Cigarette smoke causes blood vessels to spasm; increases LDL, or "bad," cholesterol; and lowers HDL, or "good," cholesterol. This results in inflammation of the cells that line the blood vessel walls and promotes blood clots. If that wasn't enough to make you quit lighting up, smoking also creates lots of cell-damaging free radicals and negates the positive effects of vitamin D_3. Needless to say, the numerous biological consequences of smoking are directly associated with heart disease and early death.

Stress

Stress results in the production of *cortisol*—the "stress" hormone—which, when produced in excess, increases blood pressure. As you know, stress can be of particular concern in African-American communities. Recent research has determined that discrimination against Blacks plays a role in their hypertension. Worries about getting a decent job, concerns about being pulled over by the police, and difficulties in getting housing can cause anxiety levels to run pretty high. Moreover, internalizing fear and anger can lead to depression and mental illness.

Fortunately, lifestyle changes such as improving your diet and incorporating exercise into your day can have a positive effect on coping with stress. This is why it is so important to consider all avenues of treatment for hypertension, not just traditional medications.

Atherosclerosis

Atherosclerosis, sometimes called hardening of the arteries, occurs when plaque—a combination of fat, cholesterol, and other substances—attaches itself to the walls of the blood vessels. As the walls of the arteries thicken with plaque, the opening of the blood vessels become narrower and harder, making it increasingly difficult for your heart to move blood throughout your body. This, in turn, raises your blood pressure and also increases your odds of suffering a heart attacks or stroke. It should be noted that hypertension itself can lead to atherosclerosis, as added pressure in blood vessels can damage the arteries, making them more vulnerable to the narrowing and plaque buildup associated with artery disease. Thus, a vicious cycle is created.

Type 2 Diabetes

Diabetes causes excessive levels of glucose (blood sugar) to flow through all blood vessels. Over time, this damages the arteries, making them targets for atherosclerosis and causing high blood pressure. As you have already read, this type of damage also increases your chance of experiencing a heart attack or stroke.

According to the American Diabetes Association, as many as two out of three diabetic adults also suffer from hypertension. Since type 2 diabetes can be effectively controlled through lifestyle changes, this is a problem that can be solved. This subject is dealt with in greater detail in Chapter 4.

Medications

While prescription drugs may be effective treatments for other conditions, certain traditional medications can actually cause hypertension. Although they are designed to reduce inflammation, corticosteroids, including prednisone and cortisone; and non-steroidal anti-inflammatory drugs (NSAIDs), including ibuprofen and aspirin, can increase blood pressure by constricting blood vessels. The same is true for migraine headache medications such as Zomig and Midrin. Tricyclic antidepressants, including amitriptyline (Elavil) and protriptyline (Vivactil), have also been known to cause hypertension over time.

Common decongestants such as pseudoephedrine (Sudafed) and diphenhydramine (Benadryl) can raise blood pressure and reduce the effectiveness of blood pressure medication. Even hormone treatments, including estrogen replacement therapy and birth control pills, have been linked to an increase in blood pressure. If you have been diagnosed with hypertension, it makes sense to discuss your medications and their side effects with your doctor.

In addition to legal medications, illegal substances, including ecstasy, cocaine, and amphetamines, can also put you at risk for high blood pressure.

HOW DO YOU REDUCE THE RISK OF HYPERTENSION?

Because of the seriousness of high blood pressure, the benefits of traditional medications to treat hypertension usually outweigh their risks. However, often, these medications do not fully resolve hypertension or the damage associated with it. That's why it makes so much sense to improve your diet, increase your activity level, and take other simple but effective steps to lower your risk of high blood pressure—steps that can also help you if you have already been diagnosed with hypertension and want to manage it.

Change Your Diet

It should come as no surprise that a healthy diet can have a tremendously positive effect not only on your blood pressure but also on your overall well-being. Little changes here and there can produce significant results that improve not only your blood pressure but also reduce your risks of the diseases associated with this condition.

By cutting your intake of alcohol, caffeine, sugar, and salt, you can reduce your body's stress level. Similarly, by avoiding an abundance of high-protein animal foods, you can decrease the anxiety-promoting compounds dopamine and norepinephrine in

MONITOR YOUR BLOOD PRESSURE AT HOME

As you are learning in this chapter, there are many steps you can take to better control your blood pressure. One of the most important things you can do is to measure your blood pressure at home. This will help you see how your blood pressure is responding to management and will also provide a valuable record for your doctor.

A blood pressure monitor may be purchased at a local pharmacy. Choose a device that has cuffs that wrap around the upper arm, as this is more accurate that devices with wrist cuffs. Get in the habit of checking your blood pressure twice a day. Keep in mind that blood pressure normally varies throughout the day, and can be affected by stress and physical activity. Be sure to measure it only after you have been sitting calmly for five minutes. Do not speak or move when checking your blood pressure.

Record your measurements in a notebook or through an app. Then take the record of your readings to appointments with your healthcare provider so that he or she can assess your progress and decide if further steps should be taken.

the brain. On the other end of the spectrum, foods that are high in complex carbohydrates and fiber can increase your levels of serotonin, the body's own calming chemical. The same can be said for eating more vegetables, which are rich in beneficial vitamins and minerals. And needless to say, decreasing your intake of high-fat foods and fried foods will help to lower your cholesterol, which can cause hypertension by resulting in plaque buildup along the walls of the blood vessels. These dietary changes can also help you fight obesity, which is also associated with high blood pressure.

The food recommendations made above are officially promoted by the National Heart, Lung, and Blood Institute through the DASH (Dietary Approaches to Stop Hypertension) diet, the American Heart Association Diet, and the Mediterranean Diet. All of these plans advocate eating fruits, vegetables, nuts, beans and legumes, and various lean meats while significantly limiting your intake of sugary beverages, fatty foods, and red meat. You can learn more about them starting on page 166 of Chapter 9.

Exercise

In addition to a healthy diet, exercise can work wonders in the battle against high blood pressure. It raises good cholesterol and lowers bad cholesterol, all the while helping you lose weight. The reduction in body mass benefits your blood pressure further by lightening the strain on your heart. Exercise also produces endorphins, which decrease stress levels. Finally, exercise lowers your blood sugar, thus helping you avoid and treat diabetes, a common cause of hypertension. So before you consider all the medications that may be prescribed to treat your hypertension, simply go for a long, brisk walk for 30 minutes per day five times per week. Create a healthy fitness routine, and those medications may never be needed. (For other exercise recommendations, see page 41 of Chapter 2.)

Quit Smoking

In addition to increasing your risk of developing high blood pressure, smoking causes heart attacks, stroke, blood clots, numerous forms of cancer, and emphysema. So much has been written about the bad health effects of smoking that I do not feel the need to say much more than this. What I will say is this: Just like the overuse of sugar and salt, smoking is an addiction. The more you smoke, the more your brain craves nicotine. And while your brain is providing you with a sense of immediate pleasure, you are literally killing all the organs in your body.

Remember that when you smoke, you are exposing your loved ones and everyone else around you to second-hand smoke, which is known to damage *their* health. If you won't quit for your own good, please quit for them. This is not to say that it's easy to quit, because it isn't. If you find that you can't do it on your own, speak to your doctor about getting some help. There are many new methods that can assist you in your goal. Cigarettes are a poison. Cut that poison out of your life.

Take Vitamin D3

As you learned earlier in the chapter, vitamin D_3 is responsible for keeping the body's production of the hormone renin in check. A deficiency in this vitamin allows an overabundance of renin, which eventually can result in high blood pressure. Taking an oral vitamin D_3 supplement can cure that deficiency, thus decreasing your chance of acquiring hypertension and the cardiovascular diseases associated with it.

Since dark-skinned people require many more times the amount of vitamin D_3 that light-skinned people require, I recommend that African Americans take between 2,000 and 5,000 IU of the supplement daily. Before starting supplementation, it's a good idea to ask your physician to order a blood test that will check your current vitamin D_3 levels. Make sure that your physician orders the 25-OH vitamin D test, which is the most accurate method available today.

Take Omega-3 Fatty Acids

Like vitamins, omega-3 and omega-6 fatty acids are required by the body for a wide range of important functions. However, the

American diet is at least ten to sixteen times too high in omega-6 fatty acids, while most Americans do not get enough omega-3s. That's unfortunate, because according to a study published in the *American Journal of Hypertension*, which examined data from 70 randomized clinical trials, omega-3 fatty acids reduce blood pressure as effectively as lifestyle changes such as exercising more and cutting back on salt. Omega-3s lower triglyceride levels, reduce inflammation, lessen the risk of blood clots, and keep the lining of the arteries smooth and free of the damage that can lead to atherosclerosis.

I encourage you to increase your consumption of fatty fish—anchovies, herring, salmon, and mackerel—as these foods are rich in omega-3s. In fact, a diet supplemented with mackerel has been reported to lower blood pressure in healthy volunteers. If you're like most people, though, you won't eat enough fatty fish to have an impact on your blood pressure. To ensure that you get the omega-3s you need, I suggest also taking supplements. The dosage of omega-3s is dependent on your individual health condition, but I recommend 1,000 mg per day for adults and 250 to 500 mg per day for children. Research has shown that omega-3 fatty acid supplements can be taken in doses up to 2,000 mg per day without side effects in adults.

Other Supplements to Consider

Along with traditional medications and well-known vitamins, other supplements have proven helpful against hypertension. Before taking any supplement, always ask your doctor if it would interfere with any medications that you're using. For guidance in choosing the best-quality supplements and using them effectively, see page 258 of A Guide to Dietary Supplements. For a more complete list of hypertension-fighting supplements, see page 271.

Folic Acid

Folic acid is a water-soluble form of vitamin B9. It is an important nutrient that the body uses to generate, replicate, and repair cells. Several studies have shown that folic acid also lowers blood pressure by relaxing and opening up the vessels, allowing for a better flow of blood. I recommend taking 400 to 500 mcg per day. Do not make the mistake of thinking that more is better. Taking too much folic acid can cause headache and diarrhea.

Hawthorn Berry

Although knowledge of this berry goes back about seven hundred years, its medicinal use was only officially recognized in 1984, when the German Commission E showed that it could lower blood pressure by opening blood vessels. It is best used by people who do not yet have hypertension, although it can supplement already established treatment. The recommended daily dosage of hawthorn berry extract is 160 to 900 mg.

Magnesium

Magnesium plays many important roles in your body. It helps send signals from your brain to all the other organs of your body, it maintains nerve cell receptors, and it is essential in generating heart muscle contractions. It also helps regulate your blood pressure by aiding the production of prostaglandin E1, a naturally occurring lipid compound that increases blood flow.

Ask your doctor to check your magnesium levels when you have your next blood test. If your levels are too low, a magnesium supplement may be beneficial. I recommend a daily dose of 400 mg to 500 mg of a time-released form of magnesium. Too much magnesium taken at once can cause unexpected bowel movements.

Coenzyme Q_{10}

Coenzyme Q_{10}, or CoQ_{10}, is an antioxidant that your body produces naturally. This nutrient aids in the body's creation of energy and is necessary for growth and maintenance. A decline in this coenzyme has major effects on the heart, decreasing the amount of energy that's available for the heart to pump efficiently and continuously.

Unfortunately, statin drugs, which are typically prescribed to combat high blood pressure, interfere with the body's production and utilization of CoQ_{10}. The body's production of this nutrient also declines naturally with age. And although this nutrient is found in meat, fish, and nuts, the amount available in these dietary sources isn't enough to sufficiently increase levels of CoQ_{10}. To compensate for any loss of this nutrient, I recommend taking CoQ_{10} supplements of up to 100 mg, one to three times a day.

CONCLUSION

Too many Americans—especially African Americans—suffer from hypertension and either don't realize that they have it or fail to take steps that can address the problem. As you now know, the result is too often a range of serious health disorders, and even a shortened life span.

Fortunately, you've also learned that you have it in your power to manage—and even eliminate—high blood pressure. By improving your diet, increasing physical activity, eliminating smoking, and using helpful dietary supplements, you can have a longer, healthier life. The more you know, the more power you have to make positive changes.

TIMELINES
FROM RECONSTRUCTION
TO THE EARLY 1900s

1865 to 1900. According to the 1870, 1880, and 1890 censuses, the death rates of African Americans during that time were staggering. They were so high, in fact, that the actuaries of New York Life Insurance Company and Equitable Holdings confidently predicted Black extinction by the year 2000. Not just poverty and poor sanitation and housing carried the "slave health deficit" way beyond the Emancipation Proclamation. Poor healthcare was also to blame. Well into the early twentieth century, most hospitals would not admit African Americans, and many White physicians refused to serve Blacks.

To combat the lack of accessibility to medical schools, schools were founded specifically for African Americans. Between 1868 and 1904, seven medical schools were established for Black students. Black physicians were denied membership in the American Medical Association, so in 1884, an all-Black medical society, the National Medical Association, was formed.

Of course, without healthcare facilities that would treat Blacks, it would be impossible for them to receive the care they needed. From 1865 to the turn of the century, each state acquired some type of healthcare facility for Black people, and by 1900, there were about forty Black hospitals. Nevertheless, healthcare for African Americans remained inadequate.

4

Diabetes

*"I chalk up the fact that I got diabetes
to my body saying, 'Dude, you have
been doing wrong for way too long!'"*
—RANDY JACKSON

What if you knew that on a certain day and time, someone was going to rob your house and injure your family members? What if you also knew which of your possessions the thief would steal, and which specific injuries would be suffered by your family? Would you take any and all preventative actions in your power to protect them? I am certain you would. Type 2 diabetes should be looked upon in the exact same way. The warning signs of the disease are known, the kind of damage it inflicts upon your body is predictable, and preventive measures can be taken to stop it. Type 2 diabetes steals your organs, your limbs, your quality of life, your finances, and finally, your life itself.

Although the primary focus of this chapter is on type 2 diabetes, the chapter begins by defining diabetes and looking at various forms of the disease. It then explores symptoms, risk factors, associated health problems, and more. Most important, it provides the tools you need to reduce the risk of this insidious disease and to help you manage it if you have already been diagnosed with the condition.

WHAT IS DIABETES?

If you look at the diagram of a cell in Figure 4.1, you'll see that when the body is healthy, a "key"—the hormone *insulin*, produced by the pancreas—unlocks an insulin receptor on the cell. This opens the glucose channel so the glucose molecules in the blood can enter the cell, where they are converted into energy. The energy is then used to fuel the body's many functions.

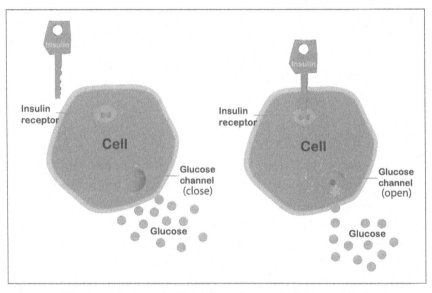

Figure 4.1. Insulin Enabling Sugar to Enter a Cell.

Diabetes is a chronic disorder in which the body is unable to produce or properly respond to insulin. This means that the glucose doesn't enter the body's cells, and the cells don't have the fuel they need to operate. Moreover, because it is not being absorbed by the cells, glucose accumulates in the bloodstream, causing numerous problems. Below, you'll learn about the various types of diabetes.

Type 1 Diabetes

In *type 1 diabetes*, once called *juvenile diabetes* or *insulin-dependent diabetes*, the pancreas secretes little or no insulin, which forces the individual to regulate his blood sugar through daily injections of the hormone. Different factors—including genetics, viruses, and perhaps other issues—contribute to type 1 diabetes. Research has found a possible connection between low levels of vitamin D and the onset of this disease, suggesting that this vitamin deficiency may allow the diabetes-causing genes to "turn on." The condition usually appears in childhood or adolescence but can also develop in adults. Although type 1 is not the focus of this chapter, the possible link between vitamin D deficiency and type 1 diabetes is worth noting.

Prediabetes

Prediabetes, also called *borderline diabetes,* is a condition in which your blood sugar is elevated but is not in the diabetes range. (See Table 4.1 on page 72.) However, over time, prediabetes can develop into type 2 diabetes if left untreated. Unfortunately, most people don't know that they are prediabetic until a doctor advises them of the condition. The symptoms, which for many are hard to recognize, can include the following:

- Blurred vision
- Fatigue
- Frequent urination
- Increased hunger
- Increased thirst
- Numbness or tingling in the fingers and arms
- Slow-healing cuts

If you are suffering from a combination of these symptoms, visit your doctor to learn if you are prediabetic.

Type 2 Diabetes

Type 2 diabetes accounts for almost 95 percent of all cases of diabetes in the United States. Unlike type 1, which occurs when the pancreas fails to produce insulin, type 2 sufferers have insulin in their bodies, but their cell membranes have become unresponsive to it, resulting in a condition called *hyperinsulinemia,* or *insulin resistance.* In other words, the body either resists the effects of insulin (the "key" doesn't quite fit in the insulin receptor or "keyhole") or doesn't produce enough insulin to maintain normal glucose levels. The main risk factors for this illness are poor diet and resulting excess weight, inactivity, inadequate sleep, and low levels of vitamin D$_3$.

Type 2 diabetes is also referred to as *adult-onset diabetes*, but in today's world, so many children are obese that they are also being diagnosed with type 2.

Gestational Diabetes

If you develop diabetes for the first time when you are pregnant, this is called *gestational diabetes*. This form of the disease puts your pregnancy at risk because babies born of mothers with gestational diabetes are often bigger. Called large-for-gestational-age babies, they can weigh 9 to 10 pounds or even more at birth. This can make it difficult for the baby to get through the birth canal and may cause the baby to experience metabolic difficulties shortly after birth.

What causes gestational diabetes? There are a number of risk factors, including overweight and obesity of the mother before pregnancy, inactivity, a previous pregnancy in which the mother had gestational diabetes, a family history of diabetes, and race. Blacks are more at risk than Whites.

Gestational diabetes also increases the risk of high blood pressure. It can cause a condition called *preeclampsia*, which is a serious complication characterized by high blood pressure, marked swelling of the hands and feet, and other problems that can threaten the lives of both mother and baby. The baby's excessive birth weight may require a Caesarian section. Babies may also be born early and have breathing complications, and are more likely to be stillborn or to die shortly after birth. Some babies have low blood sugar (hypoglycemia), which can cause seizures. Later in life, babies of mothers who had gestational diabetes are more likely to develop obesity and type 2 diabetes.

Because gestational diabetes can be so dangerous for both mother and child, it's vital to take steps to prevent it. First, eat healthy foods—fruits, vegetables, and whole grains. (See the discussion on page 81.) Second, maintain an exercise program both before and during your pregnancy. (Of course, once you become pregnant, you must consult with your healthcare provider about the exercise that's safest for you.) Third, try to start your pregnancy with a healthy weight. Fourth, try to maintain the weight increases your doctor recommends—too much weight gain increases your risk. Fifth, take your prenatal vitamins as prescribed by your doctor. Finally, be sure to keep all your appointments with your doctor so that problems are detected and treated as soon as they occur.

After birth, blood sugar usually returns to normal, but you will have a higher risk of developing type 2 diabetes later in life. And if your baby weighed more than 9 pounds, your risk of type 2 is also increased.

SYMPTOMS OF DIABETES

Unlike hypertension (high blood pressure), which rarely has any symptoms, diabetes does have symptoms. In fact, perhaps no other disease provides so many warning signs. Similar to those listed in the section on prediabetes (see page 69), they include:

- Areas of darkened skin, usually in the armpits and neck
- Blurred vision
- Fatigue
- Frequent infections
- Frequent urination
- Increased hunger
- Increased thirst
- Slow-healing sores
- Unintended weight loss

If you are experiencing any of these symptoms, immediately make an appointment with your healthcare provider.

DIAGNOSIS

Diabetes is diagnosed through a fasting blood glucose test and a hemoglobin A1c test, also known as HbA1c.

A *fasting blood glucose test* measures the level of glucose in your blood at the time of the test. Before taking this simple blood test, you can eat and drink nothing but water for at least eight hours.

A *hemoglobin A1c (HbA1c) test* is a measure of blood glucose over time. When glucose builds up in your blood, it becomes attached to hemoglobin, which is the part of the red blood cell that carries oxygen. Since red blood cells live for about ninety days, your A1c is a measure of glucose for the last two to three months.

Table 4.1 interprets the results of these two tests, showing whether they indicate no diabetes, prediabetes, or diabetes.

Table 4.1. Interpreting the Results of Fasting Glucose and Hemoglobin A1c Tests			
TEST	**No Diabetes**	**Prediabetes**	**Diabetes (type 1 or 2)**
Fasting Blood Glucose Test	Less than 100 mg/dl	Less than or equal to 100 to 125 mg/dl	Less than or equal to 126 mg/dl
Hemoglobin A1c Test	Less than 5.6%	More than or equal to 5.7 to 6.4%	More than or equal to 6.5%

RISK FACTORS

Diabetes has not only a number of distinctive symptoms, which were discussed earlier, but also a number of factors that increase your risk of getting the disease. These factors include the following.

ACANTHOSIS NIGRICANS. If you have darkened areas of skin around your neck or your armpits, this is called *acanthosis nigricans*. The darkening indicates a high level of insulin and glucose and is a very early warning sign that type 2 diabetes may develop years later. It is often seen in children years before any lab tests showing the presence of diabetes. If your children have this dark ring around the back of their necks, as if the neck is dirty, take them to their pediatrician to be checked. This would also be a good time to examine your own eating habits. It should be noted that this condition is most common in Latinos.

AGE. After age forty-five, your risk of type 2 diabetes increases. This is probably due to the greater inactivity and weight gain often associated with age.

FAMILY HISTORY. If a member of your family has type 2 diabetes, it is likely that you have a *cultural* predisposition to the disease. You see, while a family history of the disease is one of the biggest risks for acquiring it, the predisposition seems to mostly affect those following a certain lifestyle, indicating that the body's metabolism is not entirely to blame. Unfortunately, the typical Western lifestyle includes overeating and getting little physical activity—factors known to increase diabetes risk. Complicating this is a cultural style of eating that features high amounts of animal fat and salt, and low amounts of protein. Some scientists also report that there may be genetic differences between Blacks and Whites that lead African Americans to have a less efficient metabolism of glucose and a physical predisposition to diabetes.

FAT DISTRIBUTION. If you are "apple" shaped, with weight around your waist, your risk of developing diabetes type 2 goes up. If you are "pear" shaped, with weight distributed around the hips and thighs, your risk of developing diabetes type 2 goes down.

INACTIVITY. A sedentary lifestyle also contributes to type 2 diabetes. Physical activity helps you control your weight, burns up glucose, and makes your cells more sensitive to insulin so that they allow glucose to enter. Studies show a decrease in insulin sensitivity in inactive people—a group which, sadly, includes most Americans. While most of the population engages in very little physical activity on a daily basis, almost a quarter of Americans get no exercise at all. Like obesity, this problem is starting to affect children as well as adults.

METABOLIC SYNDROME. Every discussion of diabetes should mention *metabolic syndrome*, previously known as syndrome X. As opposed to the disease itself, this syndrome is a group of symptoms that precedes the onset of type 2 diabetes. The presence of three or more of the following five symptoms is required for a diagnosis of metabolic syndrome: high triglyceride levels, low HDL (good) cholesterol levels, high blood pressure, high blood glucose levels, and a waist circumference of more than 40 inches for a man or 35 inches for a woman.

OVERWEIGHT AND OBESITY. Being overweight or obese is a major risk factor for type 2 diabetes. See Chapter 2 to determine whether you are overweight or obese.

PREDIABETES OR GESTATIONAL DIABETES. Having had either of these disorders increases your risk for type 2 diabetes. (See the section beginning on page 68 for a discussion of these conditions.)

RACE. Blacks are 60 percent more likely than Whites to have type 2 diabetes. Obesity—especially if you are "apple" shaped, with weight around your waist—is a major risk factor present in so many Blacks. A lack of good healthcare, poor dietary practices, and the poverty characteristic of many Black communities also contribute to the disorder.

POOR SLEEP HABITS. According to scientists, people who get less than five hours of sleep per night are at an increased risk for type 2 diabetes. Similar to the effects of inactivity and obesity, a failure to get the recommended seven to eight hours of sleep per night can result in insulin resistance, increasing the demand on the pancreas and raising blood sugar.

VITAMIN D$_3$ DEFICIENCY. Mounting scientific evidence connects low levels of vitamin D$_3$ with diabetes and diminished control of the disease. Defects found in vitamin D receptor genes have proven to result in two genetic variants: one is linked to excessive weight gain, and the second, to impaired insulin sensitivity and low levels of "good" cholesterol. In addition, vitamin D$_3$ deficiency may cause an increase in parathyroid hormone, which promotes insulin resistance and is associated with diabetes, hypertension, inflammation, and cardiovascular disease. Research also suggests that obese children and adolescents have a higher risk of developing abnormal blood sugar when their vitamin D3 levels are low. Finally, statistics show that African Americans and Latinos display poorer control of the disease than Whites, which I suspect has much to do with the increased effort it takes for dark skin to synthesize sunlight into vitamin D3.

If you exhibit any of the above warning signs, be sure to have a conversation about type 2 diabetes with your doctor. Most important, ask that your blood glucose and HbA1c be measured. (See the discussion on page 71.)

THE EFFECTS OF DIABETES ON YOUR BODY

Both type 1 and type 2 diabetes have the same long-term destructive potential. However, even when type 1 diabetes is controlled through the use of medication, this condition slowly wreaks havoc on your system over time. Type 1 diabetes begins to damage your body—primarily your heart, brain, and kidneys—years before a diagnosis is made. That damage is mainly the result of a process called *glycation*, which eventually causes atherosclerosis and atherosclerosis-related cardiovascular disease. (You'll learn about atherosclerosis on page 76.) This, no doubt, can occur in type 2 diabetes as well, but it has a greater likelihood of being controlled with medications in type 2. Furthermore, type 2 diabetes can be cured if it is caught early enough and nutritional practices, weight, and cultural habits are modified.

Glycation happens when sugar molecules bind to proteins or fats in the body, creating harmful compounds called *advanced glycation end products*, or *AGEs*. AGEs occur naturally in everyone, but their number and rate of production are accelerated by the excess blood glucose characteristic of diabetes. AGEs impair cellular function and create free radicals, which in turn create oxidative stress, inflammation, and cell and organ damage.

It is with inflammation that we connect diabetes to cardiovascular illnesses, which can so easily take your life. Inflammation leads to a number of serious conditions, as listed below. Unfortunately, diabetes often goes hand in hand with hypertension,

THE FACTS ABOUT TYPE 2 DIABETES IN AFRICAN AMERICANS

As you now know, while diabetes affects all races, it is particularly common in the African-American community. The following facts were provided by the Office of Minority Health.

- African-American adults are 60 percent more likely than non-Hispanic White adults to be diagnosed with diabetes by a physician.

- In 2016, non-Hispanic Blacks were 3.5 times more likely to be diagnosed with end-stage renal disease when compared with non-Hispanic Whites.

- In 2016, non-Hispanic Blacks were 2 to 3 times more likely to be hospitalized for lower limb amputations when compared with non-Hispanic Whites.

- In 2017, African Americans were twice as likely as non-Hispanic Whites to die from diabetes.

which increases your risk of cardiovascular disease even further. This fact is especially problematic for the Black population, which already has extremely high rates of severe or uncontrolled high blood pressure.

The following are some of the most common disorders associated with diabetes.

ATHEROSCLEROSIS. *Atherosclerosis,* also called hardening of the arteries, is a narrowing of the arteries caused by the buildup of cholesterol-containing *plaque,* a fatty wax-like substance. The inside wall/lining of the blood vessels, irritated by inflammation caused by diabetes, becomes more easily damaged by smoking, high blood pressure, high fat levels, and high cholesterol levels, allowing plaque to build up. This can lead to strokes and heart attacks as the narrowing blood vessels cause *ischemia*—an inadequate blood supply to organs and other parts of the body.

DIABETIC RETINOPATHY. This eye condition is all too common in diabetics, causing blurred vision, distorted vision, and sometimes blindness. Poorly controlled blood sugar or many years of diabetes damage the tiny blood vessels located in the *retina,* the layer at the back of the eyeball that passes impulses to the brain, eventually resulting in a visual image. The damaged blood vessels then begin to leak fluid into the eye, causing problems. This is a progressive disorder, meaning that it gets worse over time. Sometimes, laser surgery can be used to improve the vision of people with diabetic retinopathy.

KIDNEY DISEASE. Just as high blood sugar levels damage the blood vessels in the retina, they also damage the blood vessels in your kidneys, potentially leading to kidney failure. Since diabetes often goes hand in hand with inflammation and hypertension, these conditions also contribute to kidney damage. If the damage is severe and of sufficiently long duration, kidney dialysis or a kidney transplant may be necessary.

NERVE DAMAGE. Resulting from chronic high levels of blood glucose, nerve damage—often called *diabetic neuropathy*—affects about 60 percent of people with diabetes. This disorder can cause tingling, numbness, burning, or pain in the hands and feet, gradually proceeding up the arm or leg. Nerve damage may lead to a feeling of numbness, which is dangerous, because if you can't feel damage to your toe, you may not realize that you have injured it. Reduced blood flow due to arterial damage can slow wound healing. Furthermore, bacteria thrive on high blood sugar. The combination of wounds that aren't noticed due to nerve damage, reduced blood flow, and high blood glucose can result in tissue death—*gangrene*—and the amputation of toes, feet, or legs.

You may have one or more family members or friends who have lost a limb because of raging diabetes. Tragically, Blacks are much more likely to have amputations than Whites. To prevent the need for amputation, demand an ultrasound of the affected limb. Next, request an angiogram, a test that can show the location of blocks in the arteries. Finally, a revascularization (opening of damaged blood vessels) can be performed to unblock blood vessels and restore normal blood flow.

If caught early enough and treated promptly, the disorders associated with diabetes can be controlled.

HOW DO YOU REDUCE THE RISK OF DIABETES?

Reducing your risk of diabetes is all about modifying your lifestyle. If you engage in regular physical activity, shed excess weight, and get more sleep, you will have taken three major steps towards stopping diabetes from entering your body and stealing your health.

CHECKING GLUCOSE WITHOUT FINGER STICKS

If you are diabetic, you know that you must check your blood sugar regularly. The greater the control of your blood sugar, the lower your risk for diabetes-associated health disorders. But perhaps you hate sticking your finger, so you don't check your blood glucose as often as your doctor recommends. Thanks to twenty-first-century technology, there are now a couple of devices that measure your blood glucose without fingersticks. Instead, each product includes a patch that is worn on the back of your upper arm, plus a tiny wire that goes into the top layer of your skin. The device sends your blood glucose number to a special reader or a smart phone. Studies show that these devices help people maintain and lower their A1c levels. And they may be covered by your insurance, Medicare, or Medicaid. (To see if you qualify for insurance coverage, contact your insurance provider and talk to your healthcare provider.)

First, there is the *Dexcom G6 Continuous Glucose Monitoring System*. As described above, the Dexcom includes a tiny sensor wire that is inserted under your skin using an applicator. This sensor reports your blood sugar levels to your smart phone or special reader, displaying current glucose levels as well as

You may realize that these three recommendations are interrelated. Losing weight requires exercise, and increasing exercise improves restorative sleep. Therefore, this is a triple header.

Below, you'll learn a little bit more about the three major components of diabetes prevention mentioned above. You'll also learn about other steps you can take to lower your risk of diabetes or, if you already have diabetes, to better manage it.

Get Regular Exercise

Every time you exercise, your body requires extra energy, which it gets from the glucose in your bloodstream and from the stored energy known as fat. Any brief period of physical activity will

historical trends in levels. A customizable alert system notifies you when your glucose levels go too high or too low. Dexcom has been approved for children over the age of two, and parents can monitor their child's glucose when they are out of the house or in school.

Another continuous glucose monitoring device is the *FreeStyle Libre*. This device is approved for people age eighteen and older. Although the device has a sensor that can be discreetly scanned with a compatible smart phone or a special reader, fingersticks are required for treatment decisions when you see your Check Blood Glucose symbol, if you suspect that readings may be inaccurate, or when you experience symptoms that may be due to high or low blood glucose. Unlike the Dexcom system, the Libre does not sent out alerts. However, the company offers a free fourteen-day trial period.

Speak to your healthcare provider about whether you could benefit from a continuous glucose monitoring device. Both devices require a doctor's prescription. If you decide to try one, your physician or pharmacist can help you get started. For more information on these devices, visit the US MED website listed on page 289 of the Resources section.

draw on some of the glucose, but continuous moderate exercise will raise your body's use of glucose—by all the muscles used—by twenty times the normal rate. This is how physical effort lowers your blood sugar.

Studies show that strength training, such as weight lifting, can control blood sugar to a degree, comparable to medication, while also helping you lose the excess weight that contributes to insulin resistance. In addition, *aerobic training*—which refers to any exercise that keeps your heart rate up over a prolonged period of time—not only lowers your blood glucose but also improves the circulation in your arms and legs, rids you of stress, and helps you sleep better at night.

A good exercise regimen consists of moderate physical aerobic exercise performed at least twenty minutes a day. (See page 41 of Chapter 2 for more information on aerobic activity.) This can be alternated with strength training. However, after doing strength training, make certain you give your muscles a couple of days off to recover so that they don't suffer fatigue and become prone to injury. If you've never worked with weights before, please do not engage in this activity without help. Most modern health facilities have certified trainers. I recommend that you work with one for several months to learn weight-training techniques that will reduce the likelihood of injury and enhance the results of your efforts. There will be a charge for the service of a trainer, but there will also be a charge if you have to seek medical help for injury and pain.

As with a new diet, always talk to your doctor before starting an exercise routine. If the activity is too intense, it can sometimes release stress hormones that increase the glucose level in your blood, which would result in the need for a little extra insulin after a heavy workout if you already have diabetes. A close eye on your blood sugar is always prudent.

Lose Excess Weight

Excess weight creates a vicious cycle that perpetuates type 2 diabetes. The state of being overweight causes insulin resistance in your muscles and fat tissues, which in turn forces your system

MUST YOU ABANDON TRADITIONAL FOODS?

If you were to tell your Grandma about the link between traditional Black food and diabetes, she would be saddened. These foods were passed down from generation to generation and have historical and cultural origins. Also, the wonderful women who prepared these dishes didn't know that they were contributing to the family's health problems. For these reasons, while I advise you to change your daily eating habits, I don't recommend abandoning traditional foods entirely. Instead, celebrate the meals once a year (okay, maybe twice). Make the occasion special by sharing family stories, especially stories that honor the women who developed and made the dishes. Eat traditional foods only occasionally, but never lose your connection to your family and the past.

to secrete more insulin. Increased insulin in your blood creates weight gain by altering hormonal signals to your cells and causing them to store fat—which raises your body's insulin resistance further, and so on.

The most important step you can take to lose weight is to maintain a healthful diet. That means eliminating many of the foods so common to African Americans. Fast food, refined sugar, white flour, soft drinks, and other highly sweetened beverages and desserts are all hallmarks of an unhealthy diet. Their nutritionally empty calories put stress on your system and contribute to insulin resistance. As suggested in Chapter 2, it would be beneficial to follow either the American Heart Association Diet or the Mediterranean Diet, which can help you lose weight while reaping the benefits of fresh fruits and vegetables, whole grains, lean meat, legumes, and other nutrient-packed foods. (To learn more about these diets, see Chapter 9.) Many of these foods are rich in fiber, too, which is known to lower blood glucose levels. (For more information on fiber and blood sugar, see the inset on page 83.)

Once you start making positive changes in your diet, you'll see positive changes in your weight. According to the American Diabetes Association, shedding 10 to 15 pounds can have tremendous health benefits, including lower blood sugar, reduced blood pressure, improved cholesterol levels, and less stress on your joints—not to mention the fact that you will find it easier to engage in physical activity, which, as you know, can help you shed pounds.

Some of the most encouraging information comes from the National Institutes of Health, which state that a healthy diet combined with exercise reduces your risk of developing type 2 diabetes by 58 percent. Always discuss any weight-loss regimen with your doctor, particularly if you are already diabetic, as your insulin, blood sugar, and any medications you are taking will need to be closely monitored.

If after reading this, you still don't feel motivated to commit to changing your nutritional habits, I challenge you to look at the people in your family who have type 2 diabetes, and think about what they go through because of their condition. Consider the medications they must use, the doctors' visits they endure, the time lost from work, the money spent on treatment, and their suffering, whether large or small. Doesn't it make sense to invest time and energy *now* to achieve greater health?

Get Adequate Sleep

Although diet and exercise are very important elements in the achievement of a healthy body weight and normal blood sugar levels, sleep appears to be heavily involved in the equation, as well. Sleep deprivation has been linked to insulin resistance and even obesity, with research suggesting that people who get less than seven to eight hours of sleep per night show an increased risk of acquiring type 2 diabetes. If you are already a type 2 diabetic, of course, sleep should be an even bigger priority.

There appears to be a strong link between sleep and your body's control of glucose. An insufficient amount of sleep disrupts the normal regulation of blood sugar levels that occurs during

THE IMPORTANCE OF DIETARY FIBER IN BLOOD GLUCOSE CONTROL

Dietary fiber—also known as *roughage*—is the part of plant foods that your body can't digest or absorb, but that nevertheless provides a host of health benefits. The profound effects that fiber can have on your body coupled with the ease with which it can be incorporated in your diet make it a powerful tool in the battle against diabetes.

As you learned in Chapter 1, fiber helps nourish the growth of good gut bacteria and therefore assists in maintaining a healthy microbiome. (See page 22.) This alone helps protect against diabetes. Dietary fiber also prevents and reduces the potential damage caused by type 2 diabetes by reducing blood glucose levels by an average of 10 percent. This happens, at least in part, because fiber slows the body's absorption of carbohydrates, thus preventing surges in blood sugar levels. In addition, fiber improves digestion by making stools easier to pass and induces a sense of fullness after meals, which prevents you from overeating.

Consider getting a total of 30 to 35 grams of fiber daily, which is easy to achieve if you increase your consumption of high-fiber foods such as fruits; vegetables; oat bran, oatmeal, and whole grains; dried beans; and sesame seeds. Just remember to boost your fiber intake slowly in order to avoid adverse effects such as bloating, flatulence, and cramps. Also drink plenty of water, which will help avoid constipation.

I also recommend eliminating any "white" foods from your meals, including white rice, pasta, white bread, potatoes, and sugar. All of these foods are low in fiber—in the case of white rice, bread, and pasta, the fiber has actually been removed from the grains—which results in very high levels of blood glucose. Over time, elevated glucose levels raise levels of insulin, causing your cells to lose their insulin sensitivity.

the stages of rest. Sleep also helps you maintain an appropriate weight by increasing your body's production of the protein hormone *leptin*, which suppresses appetite, and decreasing production of the hormone *ghrelin*, which stimulates appetite. This may help explain why people who get inadequate sleep are more likely to be overweight than those who get their rest.

Improve Your Microbiome

As explained in Chapter 1, a healthy microbiome (bacteria in the gut) is necessary for physical well-being. In contrast, a poor microbiome is associated with a range of serious health problems, including obesity and type 2 diabetes.

As you work to improve your diet, be sure to add probiotic foods—such as yogurt—to your daily menus and to start taking probiotic supplements. This can begin changing your microbiome within twenty-four hours. The results can include easier weight loss, as well as improvements in your immune response, lower blood pressure, and better neurological function. That's a lot of reward for very little effort! (To learn about probiotic foods and supplements, turn to page 23 of Chapter 1.)

Take Vitamin D₃

If you have read Chapter 2, you know that Vitamin D_3 is needed not only to build strong bones and teeth, but also to alleviate many health disorders. In fact, evidence suggests that adequate levels of vitamin D_3 can help you avoid type 2 diabetes and can increase your life expectancy if you already have the disease.

In one study, it was shown that those with diabetes have a much lower level of vitamin D_3. In another study, vitamin D_3 levels were linked to survival rates of patients suffering from a combination of heart disease, hypertension, type 2 diabetes, and renal failure. Those patients with the lowest levels of the nutrient had a one-year survival rate of 66 percent, while those with the highest levels had a one-year survival rate of 96 percent.

Sufficient levels of vitamin D_3 have shown the ability to improve insulin sensitivity, even in people whose blood sugar is normal. Research suggests that vitamin D_3 also plays a role in proper insulin secretion through its protective effects on *beta cells*, the pancreatic cells that produce insulin. Damage to beta cells is the reason diabetics still succumb to the ravages of the illness even when it is "under control." Clearly, the preservation of beta cells is paramount.

For anyone with a family history of type 2 diabetes, I recommend a daily 2,000 IU dose of vitamin D_3. If you already have type 1 or type 2 diabetes, I suggest increasing the dosage to 5,000 IU per day. If you have darker skin, your vitamin D_3 blood levels are generally going to be lower than the norm. In this case, you may need to double your daily dose. The best way to determine how much vitamin D_3 you require is to have your blood levels tested, and if necessary, strive to raise them to between 50 and 80 ng/mL. Make sure that your physician orders the 25-OH vitamin D test, as this will give you the best indication of your vitamin D body stores.

Consider Taking Other Supplements

In addition to vitamin D_3, there are a number of other supplements that can help you avoid or better manage type 2 diabetes by encouraging the proper metabolism of blood glucose. The following supplements have shown the most promise. For guidance in choosing the best-quality supplements and using them effectively, see the guide to supplements on page 258.

Alpha-Lipoic Acid

Alpha-lipoic acid is a potent antioxidant that helps prevent the heart and kidney damage that often accompanies diabetes. It also reduces fat accumulation and protects pancreatic beta cells, which are the cells that synthesize and secrete insulin. If you have diabetes, recommended doses of alpha-lipoic acid range from 100 to 200 mg taken three times a day. This supplement works best when used in combination with *gamma-linolenic acid*, or GLA—an omega-6 fatty acid found in plant-based oils. GLA should be taken at dosages of 400 to 600 mg per day.

Chromium Picolinate

Chromium picolinate is an essential trace mineral required for the proper metabolism of carbohydrates, fats, and proteins. It has also been shown to promote increased glucose tolerance in type 2 diabetics. According to studies, taking a daily chromium picolinate supplement of 1,000 mcg significantly improves glucose levels as well as HbA1c test levels, which are used to detect diabetes. (See page 71 for information on diabetes testing.)

Cinnamon

Researchers have determined that cinnamon contributes to a healthy glucose metabolism. A study by the US Department of Agriculture discovered that cinnamon contains water-soluble compounds called *polyphenol polymers*, which increase insulin-dependent glucose metabolism twenty fold. These compounds essentially turn on insulin-receptor genes, thereby raising glucose uptake and lowering blood glucose levels.

To take advantage of cinnamon's health benefits, add at least $1/4$ to $1/2$ teaspoon of cinnamon to your diet twice a day. You can stir it into tea or coffee or sprinkle it on toast or oatmeal. (Cold cereals are not recommended at any time.) You can also take capsules of the supplement *cinnulin,* which is cinnamon extract. A dose of 125 to 150 mg three times daily is recommended.

Coenzyme Q_{10}

A compound naturally produced in the body and also found in some foods, coenzyme Q_{10}, also called CoQ_{10}, acts as an antioxidant to prevent oxidative stress caused by free radicals, lower blood pressure, reduce cholesterol levels, and improve blood sugar control. Not surprisingly, individuals with high blood sugar, high blood pressure, and high cholesterol are often found to be deficient in this compound. Thankfully, supplementation has shown positive results.

In human trials, type 2 diabetics who were given 100 mg of CoQ_{10} twice daily showed increased blood sugar control and lower blood pressure. In another study, CoQ_{10} supplementation improved blood flow in type 2 diabetics, an outcome attributed to its ability to lower vascular oxidative stress. Finally, in animal studies, CoQ_{10} has been proven to neutralize free radicals, improve blood flow, lower triglyceride levels, and raise HDL (good) cholesterol levels, which suggests that the compound may have a role in preventing and managing complications due to diabetes.

If you are at high risk for diabetes or have been diagnosed with this disorder, I recommend that you take 100 mg of CoQ_{10} one to three times daily. Make certain you check with your healthcare provider before starting supplementation, of course.

Dehydroepiandrosterone (DHEA)

Dehydroepiandrosterone, or *DHEA,* is a naturally occurring hormone that is produced by the adrenal glands and easily converted into testosterone and estrogen. Supplementation with DHEA is known to improve insulin sensitivity in type 2 diabetics, who tend to have low levels of the hormone. Although the mechanisms behind this improvement aren't fully understood, it has been suggested that DHEA's conversion to testosterone may be responsible, as testosterone raises insulin sensitivity. Research into DHEA has also shown a potential benefit of supplementation for type 1 diabetics, as the hormone seems to increase pancreatic beta cells in animals. Other advantages of supplementation include the hormone's ability to produce antioxidant enzymes in the liver, reduce fat tissue, relieve stress, strengthen the immune system, maintain sexual desire, and improve mental clarity. It should be noted that DHEA levels are highest when you are about twenty years old and decline significantly as you age.

The dosage of DHEA depends on a number of variables, including your height, weight, gender, and even your stress level. I recommend that women start with 25 mg per day, and men, with 50 to 100 mg per day. If possible, get your DHEA level checked to give you a better idea of the amount that is appropriate for you. Because DHEA can cause high levels of testosterone and estrogen, anyone with a history of breast or prostate cancer should discuss the use of this compound with a doctor before beginning supplementation.

Green Tea Extract

Green tea contains an abundant amount of *catechins*, which fall into the family of polyphenols previously discussed in connection with cinnamon. These compounds are powerful antioxidants that are particularly effective at ridding the pancreas and liver of toxins. Animal studies have shown that the catechins found in green tea may play a role in the prevention of diabetes by stopping the destruction of beta cells. Finally, lab studies suggest that green tea may suppress diet-induced obesity.

I recommend adding 6 to 9 drops of green tea extract to 32 ounces of water and drinking the mixture throughout the day.

Selective Kinase Receptor Modulators (SKRMs)

Medical breakthroughs are occurring in an area that may be new to you: medical food. As defined by the Food and Drug Administration, a medical food is "a food which is formulated to be consumed or administered . . . under the supervision of a physician and which is intended for the management of a disease or condition for which distinctive nutritional requirements, based on recognized scientific principles, are established by medical evaluation." These foods are called *selective kinase receptor modulators*, or *SKRMs* (pronounced skirm), because they affect enzymes called *kinases*, which activate or inhibit various molecules, including proteins, fats, and carbohydrates. Up to 518 different kinases have been identified in humans.

With this in mind, researchers are in search of foods that can target selected kinases and modulate them in an attempt to alter the course of diseases such as type 2 diabetes. Two of the most promising foods are hops and acacia, which have been utilized medicinally in certain cultures for centuries. These plants support healthy blood sugar and triglyceride levels, and thus may be recommended to patients who have been diagnosed with metabolic syndrome or type 2 diabetes. *Insinase*, a nutritional supplement that has been designed to improve glucose metabolism, contains both of these naturally occurring SKRMs. Talk to your healthcare provider to see if medical food supplements would benefit your condition.

CONCLUSION

Type 2 diabetes is a progressive illness that slowly destroys your body if it isn't controlled by changes in lifestyle and by medication. This disorder is caused by a number of factors, including weight gain, lack of exercise, and poor sleep, as well as inadequate levels of vitamin D_3. Moreover, an insufficiency of certain nutrients, hormones, and other substances may play a part in the development of diabetes.

Although type 2 diabetes is having devastating effects on the African-American community, it is a controllable disease because the factors that contribute to it are modifiable. Weight loss, regular physical activity, and sufficient rest can decrease the risk of acquiring type 2 diabetes and may potentially reverse its symptoms should you already be affected by the illness. These three lifestyle tactics work best in concert, with each boosting the effectiveness of the other. Exercise helps you lose weight and sleep better, while more sleep aids in weight loss, making it easier for you to exercise. Additionally, by maintaining an adequate level of vitamin D_3, you can improve insulin sensitivity in your body and prevent the loss of pancreatic beta cells. If you also add a few of the supplements mentioned in this chapter to your daily routine, you can build a strong defense against type 2 diabetes.

The most important thing to realize is that a diagnosis of this illness is not irreversible. If you pay attention to the early signs of type 2 diabetes and make important lifestyle changes, you can return your body to a healthy state and avoid the complications associated with this all-too-common disease. The knowledge provided in this chapter has empowered you to take charge of your health.

TIMELINES
THE GREAT MIGRATION

1915 to 1960. There came a time when the post-Civil War anti-Black Jim Crow laws of the South became unbearable for African Americans. Allowed to work in only the most menial jobs and denied basic civil rights, such as the right to vote, they lived in grinding poverty, with little hope for improvement. For this reason, between 1915 and 1960, over 5 million Black Americans moved from the Deep South states of South Carolina, Georgia, Louisiana, Mississippi, and Alabama to the northern cities of Chicago, Cleveland, Detroit, New York City, Philadelphia, and Washington, DC, searching for a better life.

It might seem that the Great Migration, with the potential of higher-paying jobs and an escape from Jim Crow laws, would deliver improved health for Black Americans, but this was not to be. Remarkably, health conditions worsened. As described in a 2015 article entitled *The Impact of the Great Migration on Mortality of African Americans*, although the Great Migration inspired hope for a better life, health problems were probably exacerbated by increased stress due to separation from families and communities; uncertainty about finding jobs, adequate housing, and a community that would provide support; a higher exposure to environmental hazards in big industrialized cities; and changing habits related to smoking, drinking alcohol, and diet. In the end, the Great Migration actually increased disease among the African Americans involved and decreased longevity.

5

Cardiovascular Disease

"The greatest miracle on Earth is the human body. It is stronger and wiser than you may realize, and improving its ability to self-heal is within your control."
—DR. FABRIZIO MANCINI

Cardiovascular disease (CVD) consistently remains the leading cause of death in the United States. Worse still, nearly 48 percent of Black women and 44 percent of Black men have some form of heart disease, and Blacks are much more likely to die of heart disease than Whites. Add to that, younger Blacks are now showing signs of CVD. But it doesn't have to be this way. CVD is both preventable and, as you will learn, in most cases reversible.

In this chapter, we will be looking at what cardiovascular disease is, what causes it, and how you can reduce your risks. The more you know about CVD, the more likely that you will be able to identify the telltale signs and take steps to improve your health.

WHAT IS CARDIOVASCULAR DISEASE?

Cardiovascular disease is essentially any health problem related to the heart and the circulatory system, which includes the veins, arteries, and capillaries.

The heart is a hollow muscular organ that uses rhythmic contractions to pump the blood throughout the circulatory system,

SYMPTOMS OF STROKE OR HEART ATTACK

Knowing the symptoms of a stroke or heart attack can save the life of a loved one, as it will enable you to get that person to the hospital for immediate treatment.

To help people easily remember the symptoms of stroke, experts have come up with the acronym BE FAST:

B: Balance. You suddenly have trouble with your balance.

E: Eyes: Your vision changes quickly and dramatically.

F: Facial droop: One side of your face gets lower than the other.

A: Arms: You cannot hold up or raise one arm.

S: Speech: Your speech changes suddenly and is garbled, slurred, or absent.

T: Time: If you have one of these symptoms, it's time to call 911 *immediately*. Don't wait!

In today's world, medical science has ways to dissolve your clot or stop hemorrhaging, but you must get treatment as soon as possible. Time is important if you are to recover and avoid permanent damage.

bringing oxygen and nutrients to the body and carrying away waste products. When that muscle begins to have problems, it is the start of cardiovascular disease. The most common heart problems include the following:

- Inflammation or infection of the heart.
- Weakening or irregularity of the heart rhythm.
- A rupture in the heart.
- A weakening of the heart.
- The formation of clots that cause blockage.

Common symptoms of heart attack include the following:

- Chest pain, which usually starts slowly and builds.
- Chest discomfort or pressure that feels like "fullness" or squeezing.
- Pain or discomfort in areas above the waist, such as the back, the upper part of the stomach, the shoulders, or even the jaws and teeth.
- Shortness of breath.
- Nausea and vomiting.
- Coughing or wheezing.
- Dizziness.

Unlike strokes, where symptoms develop quickly, the warning signs of a heart attack often start with mild discomfort that lasts thirty minutes or longer. The most common symptom for both men and women is chest pain or discomfort. But women are more likely than men to experience some of the other common symptoms, particularly shortness of breath, nausea and vomiting, and back or jaw pain.

When you suspect a heart attack, you must call 911 immediately to get prompt treatment that reduces damage to the heart muscle. Fast action can save lives—maybe even your own.

The circulatory system has its own set of problems, which include:

- Inflammation or infection of the blood vessels.
- Hardening of the veins and arteries.
- Narrowing of the blood vessels.
- Blockage of the blood vessels.
- Bulging or ballooning of the blood vessels.
- Formation of clots in the blood vessels.

Each of these conditions has a medical name along with symptoms, diagnosis, likely outcome if left untreated, and treatments. If a condition is allowed to progress without medical management, the result can be high blood pressure, a lost body part due to lack of circulation, heart attack, stroke, and possibly even death.

While there is a small chance that some of these conditions are genetic, for the vast majority of people suffering from CVD, the risk factors are directly tied to lifestyle choices. And based on the statistics, we are definitely doing something wrong. You will learn more about the causes of CVD below.

THE CAUSES OF CARDIOVASCULAR DISEASE

There are a number of risk factors that make cardiovascular disease more likely to occur. They include the following:

- Cigarette smoking
- Diabetes
- High cholesterol and triglycerides
- Hypertension
- Overweight and obesity
- Poor diet

In many cases, these risk factors are tied together. A heavy smoker who is overweight; a diabetic with high blood pressure; or a person who is heavy, has a junk food diet, and is under a lot of stress—all of these individuals are more likely than the average person to develop cardiovascular disease. And while all of these risk factors are easy to spot, too few people do anything to change them until it's too late.

In today's world, there is an app for just about everything—even for determining your risk of stroke. To learn more, see the inset on page 95.

Cigarette Smoking

How bad is cigarette smoke? Consider this: If I were to take all the toxic chemicals found in cigarette smoke and deliberately place them in the food you eat and the liquid you drink, and you could prove that I did it, I could be charged with attempted murder. And if you died because of what I had done, the charge would be upgraded to premeditated murder. Why would you willingly expose yourself to these same chemicals?

If this hasn't convinced you that smoking is bad, consider this: Smoking is a major cause of cardiovascular disease and causes one out of every four deaths from CVD. Smoking can:

- Raise triglyceride levels.

- Lower "good" HDL cholesterol.

- Make blood sticky and more likely to clot, which can block blood flow to the heart and brain.

- Damage the cells that line the blood vessels.

- Increase the buildup of plaque in the blood vessels.

- Cause thickening and narrowing of blood vessels (atherosclerosis).

STROKE RISKOMETER

If you want a quick and easy way to determine your risk of stroke, try a free app that is now available on smart phones and tablets. Endorsed by the World Stroke Organization, the Stroke Riskometer can inform you of your risk of having a stroke in the next five or ten years. Keep in mind that if you are at risk for stroke, you are at an even greater risk for heart attack.

All you have to do is answer twenty questions about your age, height, weight, family history, blood pressure, and so on. Based on your answers, the app will calculate your personal risk. It will also show you how your risk level compares with that of someone of the same age who has no risk factors. Visit the website www.strokeriskometer.com to learn more about this valuable app.

If you combine smoking with being overweight, lack of exercise, poor nutrition, hypertension, or diabetes, your body is a ticking time bomb ready to go off. And when it does explode, it's likely to be in the form of a heart attack, a stroke, or death.

Diabetes

Diabetes and hypertension are like the Blues Brothers: They very often travel together causing trouble. As explained in Chapter 4, when diabetes prevents you from controlling the amount of glucose (sugar) in your blood, the resulting high glucose levels injure the interior of the blood vessel walls. Unregulated glucose along with high blood pressure—which also injures blood vessels—begins the cascade of events that lead to CVD, greatly increasing your odds of dying before your time. The longer you have diabetes, the greater your chances of developing heart disease. People with diabetes also tend to develop heart disease at a younger age than people who do not have diabetes. (For more information on diabetes and its management, see Chapter 4.)

High Cholesterol and Triglycerides

Both cholesterol and triglycerides are lipids (fats) that are naturally present in the body. Cholesterol is consumed in food and is also made by the liver. The body also manufactures triglycerides. Although neither of these substances is inherently bad, when they are present in large amounts, they can lead to cardiovascular

Table 5.1. Ideal Cholesterol and Triglyceride Levels	
Type of Cholesterol	**Ideal Level (mg/dL)**
Total Cholesterol	Less than 200
LDL Cholesterol	Less than 70
HDL Cholesterol	Men: Over 40; Women: Over 50
Triglycerides	Less than 150

disease by forming plaque deposits on the inside of the arteries, thereby slowing or blocking blood flow. To learn more about cholesterol and triglycerides, see the inset on page 98.

Hypertension

If you read Chapter 3, you know that hypertension, or high blood pressure, can lead to atherosclerosis by damaging the arteries and making them more vulnerable to the narrowing and plaque deposits associated with this disease. Hypertension also forces your heart to work harder to pump your blood throughout your body. This causes part of your heart—the left ventricle—to thicken, increasing your risk of heart attack, heart failure, and sudden cardiac death.

African Americans are more likely to have high blood pressure than their white counterparts, and many people don't even know they have it. Remember that hypertension is called the "silent killer" because there are no obvious symptoms to tell you it's there. This is why it's so important to get annual checkups and, if you are diagnosed with high blood pressure, to take steps to control it. (For more information on hypertension and its management, see Chapter 3.)

Overweight and Obesity

As discussed in Chapter 2, obesity increases the risk of high cholesterol and triglyceride levels and diabetes—both of which make it more likely that you will develop coronary heart disease. Obese individuals also require more blood to supply oxygen and nutrients to the body, which causes an increase in blood pressure. And as you learned in this chapter, high blood pressure also increases the risk of heart disease. The link between obesity and cardiovascular disease makes it vitally important to control your weight. (For more information on obesity and its management, see Chapter 2.)

Poor Diet

You are probably already aware that the foods we eat affect our health. But you may not know that researchers who analyzed data from the National Health and Nutrition Examination Survey found that every year, *almost half of deaths* (about 45 percent) from heart disease, stroke, and type 2 diabetes can be linked to a poor diet.

The greatest number of deaths from heart disease were associated with a high consumption of sugar-sweetened beverages and processed meats as well as a low intake of nuts. High stroke risk was found to be associated with a diet high in salt but low in fruits and vegetables. Increased death from diabetes was linked with eating a large amount of processed meats and sugar-sweetened drinks, and a low amount of whole grains.

The study illustrates that the choices you make every time you eat can have a profound impact on your overall health and on cardiovascular wellness.

CHOLESTEROL, TRIGLYCERIDES, AND CARDIOVASCULAR DISEASE

Almost everyone thinks that *cholesterol*—a waxy lipid (fat) that circulates in the blood—is bad. But it's like blood glucose: You must have the right amount, but not too much! After all, some cholesterol is required by the body to make your sex and stress hormones. Cholesterol is also needed to build cells and to make vitamin D_3.

A problem occurs when there is too much cholesterol circulating in the body, and especially when you have too much of the wrong type of cholesterol. You probably know that when your healthcare provider orders a Lipid Profile, he checks not only for total cholesterol but also for LDL and HDL cholesterol. LDL stands for *low-density lipoprotein*, and HDL stands for *high-density lipoprotein*. LDL is often called "bad" cholesterol because it takes cholesterol to your arteries, where it can collect on artery walls in the form of plaque. HDL is often called "good" cholesterol because it removes excess cholesterol from your body. You want the LDL to

WHAT ARE THE MAJOR PROBLEMS ASSOCIATED WITH CARDIOVASCULAR DISEASE?

In our discussion of risk factors, we mention several major cardiovascular problems that can occur, such as heart attack and stroke. While people often use these terms, too many don't really understand what they are. The following discussions provide basic information about some of the most common forms of cardiovascular disease.

Heart Attack

A *heart attack* occurs when the flow of blood in one or more of the coronary arteries that supply the heart muscle suddenly become blocked, and a section of the heart can't get the oxygen it needs. The blockage is usually caused when plaque—fatty deposits on the

be low, and the HDL to be high. When your HDL is high, your LDL is low, and your total cholesterol is low, you're in good shape.

In addition to measuring cholesterol, a Lipid Profile also measures *triglycerides.* Like cholesterol, triglycerides are a type of lipid. When you eat, your body converts the calories it doesn't immediately need into triglycerides, which are stored in your fat cells. Later, triglycerides are released for energy as needed between meals.

The role that triglycerides play in heart disease is not as clear as the role played by cholesterol. However, it is known that this substance increases inflammation in the blood vessels. It is also known that when inflammation is present and your total cholesterol or LDL levels are high, you are at increased risk for atherosclerosis, or hardening of the arteries. Moreover, recent research has concluded that triglycerides alone have a big impact on mortality risk for patients with heart disease. This is why it's so important to maintain low levels of both cholesterol and triglycerides.

What are considered ideal cholesterol and triglyceride levels? Table 5.1 on page 96 presents the best levels. Keep them in mind the next time your doctor reviews your Lipid Profile test with you.

lining of the blood vessels—ruptures (breaks open), leading to the formation of a blood clot. If the clot becomes large enough, it can partially or completely block the coronary artery. The decreased blood flow causes a decrease in the amount of oxygen that flows to those tissues. Without oxygen, the heart muscle can no longer do its work, which is to pump blood to the body and itself. If the blockage isn't treated quickly enough, the portion of the heart supplied by the artery can die.

A heart attack, therefore, is not when the heart stops, although that can and does occur. It is an injury to the heart. This injury may also cause the heart to beat differently so that your blood cannot be pumped effectively through your body.

People who survive this event may recover, but if the heart cannot be repaired by medication, surgery, or lifestyle changes, they may be permanently disabled. Don't wait for a heart attack to occur. You don't want to be one of the numbers adding to the yearly statistic of Blacks dying from CVD.

Other Heart Problems

There are many other problems that can affect your heart. In the following discussion, I will cover just two. Both are common and can lead to stroke.

Atrial Fibrillation

Atrial fibrillation occurs when the two upper chambers of the heart, known as the atria, receive chaotic electrical signals. When this happens, the atria do not squeeze properly, but instead quiver, causing a fast and irregular heart rhythm. As a result, blood is more likely to remain stagnant, or pool, in the atria, leading to the formation of clots. If a clot dislodges, it can be thrown into the arteries leading to the brain, causing an ischemic stroke (see the section on strokes that begins on page 101). Untreated, atrial fibrillation increases the risk of stroke by a factor of approximately five. Blood-thinning drugs such as warfarin can reduce the risk of ischemic stroke due to atrial fibrillation by making it less likely for a clot to form in the heart.

Atrial fibrillation often does not cause any symptoms. When it does, patients often report that they feel their hearts pounding or "flip-flopping" in their chests. They may also complain of fatigue, generalized weakness, decreased exercise endurance, dizziness, and shortness of breath. If you experience these symptoms, be sure tell your healthcare provider immediately so that treatment can begin. Always take your medicine as directed, and don't stop when you begin to feel better!

Heart Failure

Despite its name, the term heart failure, also called congestive heart failure, does not mean that the heart is not working. Instead, *heart failure* is a chronic, progressive condition in which the heart works less effectively than normal because one or more chambers of the heart "fail" to keep up with the volume of blood flowing through them. As a result, blood moves through the heart and body at a slower rate, and the heart cannot pump enough oxygen and nutrients to meet the body's needs. When the heart doesn't pump efficiently, the blood in the heart becomes prone to forming clots, which can be delivered to the brain, causing a stroke. Heart failure has several causes, the most common being high blood pressure and heart attack. Other causes include damaged heart valves, infection or inflammation of the heart muscle, excessive use of alcohol, type 2 diabetes, obesity, and high cholesterol.

Heart failure can cause numerous symptoms, including fatigue, weight gain, shortness of breath, increased urination at night, low energy, and swelling of the leg, ankle, or foot. If you have these symptoms and have been diagnosed with heart failure, ask your healthcare provider what you can do to reduce your risk of stroke.

Stroke

A stroke is similar to a heart attack but occurs in the brain. There are three types of strokes. The most common type is the *ischemic stroke*, which is usually caused by a blood clot that prevents blood from getting to the brain. When this occurs, brain cells, deprived of blood, begin to die very quickly.

COMMON MYTHS ABOUT CARDIOVASCULAR DISEASE

Unfortunately, there are many myths about cardiovascular disease, and some of these myths may keep you from making important health-restoring changes in your life. Below, I will dispel some of these falsehoods.

I'm likely to get a heart attack or a stroke when I feel my blood pressure increasing.
Wrong. You won't know if your BP is elevated, which is why we call hypertension a "silent killer." If you do have hypertension, the stroke or heart attack is going to surprise you—that is, if you survive it. The unfortunate fact is that 70 percent of those who experience these events do *not* survive them. I'm not trying to scare you. I'm simply stating the facts.

I'm too young to get cardiovascular disease, so I don't have to worry about it.
Wrong. If you are a smoker, are overweight, have high blood pressure, or have high cholesterol, you are not too young to have heart disease. Begin taking steps to manage your conditions and to improve your cardiovascular health.

The second type of stroke is the *hemorrhagic stroke,* which occurs when a weakened blood vessel bursts and bleeds into the surrounding brain. Pressure from the leaked blood damages the brain cells, and the damaged area is unable to function properly.

Another type of stroke is a *transient ischemic attack,* or *TIA.* This occurs when the supply of blood to an area of the brain is blocked but then restored. As its name implies, a TIA is temporary, and damage is not sustained. Even though the symptoms of a TIA subside, it is critical to go to the hospital after experiencing one to determine why it happened and to start medications to prevent another stroke. In some cases, an urgent intervention such as surgery may be indicated. The short-term risk of having a stroke

These conditions have been in my family forever, so I can't escape them.

Wrong. As I emphasize throughout this book, no matter the statistics or even your family history, you can improve your physical well-being and avoid cardiovascular disease. And before you decide that the problem is genetic, look at what your family eats and what their habits are. Do they eat high-fat, low-nutrition foods? Are they overweight? Do they smoke? Do they rarely if ever exercise? By making good lifestyle choices, you can overcome genetic disadvantages and enjoy a long and healthy life.

When I get chest pain, is that a heart attack?

You can't tell. However, if you have diabetes, are overweight, have high cholesterol/triglycerides, and/or smoke, don't wait and play guessing games. Call your healthcare provider and get checked out. If your healthcare provider isn't available, go to the nearest emergency room.

If you have chest pain but have none of the conditions mentioned above, very likely, you have indigestion, which can mimic the symptoms of a heart attack. But if the symptoms are painful and last for more than a few minutes, you should definitely contact your healthcare provider. If it turns out to be a heart attack, it's vital to get immediate treatment.

after a TIA is as high as 10 percent at two days, and 17 percent at ninety days.

Since different part of your brain control different activities—speaking, walking, thinking, etc.—the type of damage caused by a stroke depends on the location of the injury to the brain. If it's serious, it may result in slurred speech or no ability to speak at all. It can cause paralysis in any or all of your limbs, or you can be in a vegetative state, meaning that you are alive but unable to respond to the outside world. Or it can kill you. Less serious strokes can lead to a number of physical and emotional issues. However, with physical therapy and appropriate medications, these problems can be overcome. As explained in the inset on page 92, if you or someone you love is showing the symptoms of having a stroke, it is vital to get to the hospital right away so that further damage can be avoided and treatment can begin.

HOW DO YOU REDUCE YOUR RISK OF CARDIOVASCULAR DISEASE?

This chapter has mentioned a number of factors that increase the risks of cardiovascular disease, including hypertension, being overweight or obese, eating a poor diet, and more. This is actually good news, because it means that you can do a great deal to improve your general health and prevent disorders of the heart and blood vessels. The following sections will point you in the right direction. If you have already been diagnosed with a cardiovascular disorder and are receiving medical treatment, be sure to speak to your healthcare provider before making a lifestyle change or taking a supplement. More than likely, though, your doctor will be enthusiastic about your efforts to end bad habits and adopt a healthier lifestyle.

Exercise

Numerous studies have shown that exercise decreases the chance of having a heart attack or experiencing another cardiac event, such as a stroke. Regular exercise promotes weight loss, helps reduce blood pressure, can lower the levels of "bad" cholesterol in the blood, and can raise the levels of "good" cholesterol. In people with diabetes, regular activity improves the body's ability to control blood glucose levels. Exercise is particularly effective when combined with other lifestyle changes, such as good nutrition and smoking cessation. If a cardiac event, such as a heart attack, has already occurred, exercise can speed recovery.

In 1996, the Surgeon General's Report on Physical Activity and Health stated that the cardiovascular benefits mentioned above will generally occur by engaging in at least thirty minutes of modest activity on most, preferably all, days of the week. Modest activity is defined as any activity that is similar in intensity to brisk walking at a rate of about three to four miles per hour. To learn more about exercise, see page 39 of Chapter 2.

Quit Smoking

Earlier in the chapter, you learned the many ways in which smoking contributes to heart disease. It is no exaggeration to say that quitting smoking is one of the most important things you can do to avoid heart attack and stroke as well as milder cardiovascular disorders.

An understanding of the relationship between smoking and heart disease may be all that you need to stop puffing on those cigarettes. But if you can't quit on your own, by all means, speak to your healthcare provider about getting help. There are many products, from patches to pills, that can help you reach your goal.

Change Your Diet

A healthy diet is one of the most important weapons in your fight against cardiovascular disease. Earlier in the chapter, you learned that heart disease and stroke have been associated with an excessive intake of sugar-sweetened drinks and processed meats, and with an inadequate consumption of nuts and grains. So how do you choose a diet that will prevent cardiovascular disease? The American Heart Association states that a heart-healthy eating plan should include the following foods:

- A variety of fruits and vegetables
- Whole grains such as brown rice, whole wheat products, and quinoa
- Low-fat dairy products
- Skinless poultry and fish
- Nuts and legumes

In addition to incorporating the foods listed above, your diet should limit saturated fat, trans fat, sodium (salt), red meat and processed meats, sweets, and sugar-sweetened beverages.

If you need help in creating a diet that includes heart-healthy foods and omits foods that have been associated with disease, you'll be glad to know that several diets can be helpful, including the DASH Diet (Dietary Approaches to Stop Hypertension), the American Heart Association Diet, and the Mediterranean Diet. These diets—especially when paired with exercise—can also help you lose excess weight. You can learn more about these diets by turning to Chapter 9 (see page 166). Page 285 of the Resources section can direct you to websites that provide guidelines for each eating plan.

Take Omega-3 Fatty Acids

In Chapter 3, which focused on hypertension, you learned that omega-3 fatty acids lower triglyceride levels, reduce inflammation, lessen the risk of blood clots, and keep the lining of the arteries smooth and free of the damage that can lead to atherosclerosis. Clearly, omega-3s can do a great deal to maintain or improve your heart health.

One of the ways in which you get more omega-3s is to eat fatty fish such as anchovies, herring, salmon, and mackerel, which are rich in this nutrient. Also add nuts to your diet. But because it's hard to get all the omega-3s that you need from food, I also suggest taking supplements. Between 1,000 and 2,000 mg per day of omega-3 fatty acids will help protect your heart in many ways.

To learn about additional supplements that can improve cardiovascular health, turn to page 267.

CONCLUSION

Although heart disease is now the leading cause of death in the United States, this statistic isn't written in stone. By adopting a healthy lifestyle—with adequate exercise, good nutrition, no smoking, and other beneficial habits—you can help keep your blood pressure, cholesterol, and blood sugar levels under control and lower your risk for heart disease, heart attack, and stroke. Now that you know the good, the bad, and the ugly about cardiovascular disorders, you can take charge of your health and your life.

TIMELINES
TWENTIETH-CENTURY EXPERIMENTS

1932 to 1972. In 1932, the US Public Health Service, working with the Tuskegee Institute, initiated the "Tuskegee Study of Untreated Syphilis in the Negro Male." It recruited 339 Black males with syphilis and 201 who did not have the disease. Of course, the participants were never told what the study was focused on, nor were they given informed consent forms. They were told they were being treated for "bad blood." For "payment," the men received free medical exams, free meals, and burial insurance. They were treated with toxic chemicals such as mercury and bismuth, and they never received adequate treatment.

At that time, there was no known cure for syphilis. The symptoms of syphilis would start with a rash and then spread to the brain, nerves, eyes, heart, and other organs. Finally, the disease would cause dementia and death. By 1947, penicillin became the drug of choice to treat syphilis effectively, but the men were never properly treated with this drug.

After a 1972 Associated Press story exposed the study, a government panel was appointed to review the Tuskegee Study. One month later, the panel advised that the study be ended. By that time, 28 men in the study had died of syphilis, 40 wives had contracted it, and it had been passed on to 19 children at birth. Unfortunately, these numbers were probably a reflection of only the most recent participants. The actual numbers were likely to have been much greater.

1942 to 1945. During World War II, the United States military believed that toxic chemicals would be used as major weapons as they had been in World War I. To better understand the reactions to these chemicals, the Army conducted secret experiments, testing the effects of exposure to mustard gas and other toxic chemicals. Thousands of US troops were involved, and in at least nine studies, the servicemen were singled out based on race. African-American, Puerto Rican, and Japanese-American troops were specifically exposed so that researchers could note their physical reactions. The purpose of the experiments was to discover if different races tolerated mustard gas better than others. According to veteran Rollins Edwards, soldiers were told that "they were being tested to see what effect these gases would have on black skins."

Supposedly, the men were "volunteers," but subsequent interviews after the war revealed that they were compelled to participate without knowledge of the known effects of chemical weapons. Mustard gas causes irreversible damage to the skin, resulting in sores that never heal and even skin cancer. It can also cause severe respiratory problems, such as COPD, emphysema, and asthma, as well as leukemia and eye disease. It was not until the 1990s that these experiments were made public.

From 1948 to 1975, the U.S. Army Chemical Corps conducted further classified human subject research at the Edgewood Arsenal facility in Maryland involving around 7,000 troops. Because these experiments are still classified, little is known about the soldiers who were used.

6

Kidney Disease

*"I'd like people to know that you can head off kidney disease,
maybe prevent a transplant or stop the disease from progressing
after detection by doing a simple urine test in the doctor's office."*
—SEAN ELLIOTT

ccording to the National Kidney Foundation, Black Americans are four times more likely to fall victim to kidney disease than White Americans. They also develop the condition at an earlier age than White Americans. And although African Americans make up only about 13 percent of the country's population, we account for a staggering 35 percent of kidney failure patients. In this chapter, we will see that many of the risk factors of kidney disease are directly linked to other conditions that are covered in this book.

First, it is important to understand how these factors are connected to the diseases that have come to plague our neighborhoods. By neglecting one illness, you may be allowing another to develop. Second, it is vital to recognize the early signs of kidney disease so that you can take action. The progression of kidney disease can be stopped in its tracks once you know what to look for and what to do. Hopefully, the following information will help you do just that.

WHAT DO THE KIDNEYS DO?

Located just below the middle of the back, one on either side of the spine, the kidneys perform numerous important functions in the body. Perhaps their most commonly known purpose is the filtration of blood and the subsequent removal of waste products, which make their way to the bladder and get excreted through urination. (See Figure 6.1 on page 112.) You see, each of your kidneys is composed of about a million filtering units cause *nephrons*, each of which includes a filter, called a *glomerulus*, and a *renal tubule*, which returns needed substances to the blood and removes waste. But the kidneys do so much more than that. These vital organs:

- Help control your blood pressure.

- Maintain your internal acid-base balance.

- Maintain a stable balance of chemicals, such as salts and other substances, in the blood.

- Produce several hormones, such as vitamin D_3 (calcitriol); renin, which is involved in blood pressure control; and erythropoietin, which plays a key role in the creation of red blood cells.

WHAT IS KIDNEY DISEASE?

Chronic kidney disease (CKD) is characterized by a gradual decrease in kidney function, which in turn can cause a host of health problems, including the accumulation of waste products (such as urine, proteins, and sodium) in the body; high blood pressure; acidosis (excess acid in the body); and anemia (deficiency of red blood cells). This can lead to various symptoms, some of which are easily recognizable in early stages. They include:

- Decreased energy.
- Difficulty sleeping.
- Dry skin.
- Foamy urine.
- Frequent urination during the night.

- High blood pressure.
- Inability to concentrate.
- Loss of appetite.
- Muscle cramps.
- Presence of blood in the urine

● Puffiness around the eyes.   ● Swelling of the ankles and
                                    legs.

Many of these symptoms are also associated with other disorders, some of which—like obesity, hypertension, and diabetes—have been discussed in previous chapters. If you find yourself experiencing any of these symptoms, make an appointment to see your healthcare provider, who will probably order a blood and/ or urine test. Don't waste your time playing guessing games. It's important to act as quickly as possible. Your healthcare provider may rule out kidney problems or may advise you to make a few changes in your life.

The Stages of Kidney Disease

There are five stages of kidney disease. Each stage is based on the individual's *glomerular filtration rate (GFR)*, which measures how well the kidneys are filtering the blood. The lower the GRF, the more serious the kidney disease. This is shown in Table 6.1, which states the GFR and level of function for each stage of the disorder.

Table 6.1. The Five Stages of Chronic Kidney Disease		
Stage of Kidney Disease	GFR	Level of Function
Stage 1	90 or higher	Kidneys show some damage but still function normally.
Stage 2	89 to 60	Kidneys show a mild loss of function.
Stage 3	59 to 30	Loss of kidney function has increased from mild to moderate.
Stage 4	29 to 15	Kidneys have a severe loss of function.
Stage 5	Less than 15	Kidneys have lost nearly or all function.

After deteriorating over a number of years, the kidneys can eventually stop working completely or nearly completely. Individuals whose kidneys have 10 percent or less of their normal ability are considered to be in *end-stage renal disease (ESRD)*, or *stage 5*. These individuals require dialysis, which is the cleaning (filtering) of toxins out of the blood using an external machine. Alternatively, a person in stage 5 can get a kidney transplant from a donor.

WHAT CAUSES KIDNEY DISEASE?

The causes of chronic kidney disease are many. While it can be inherited—as in the case of polycystic kidney disease—or can result

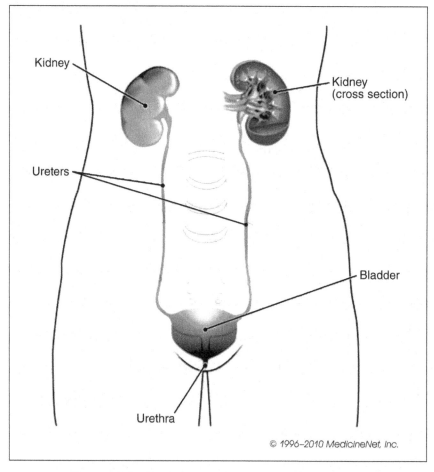

Figure 6.1. The Path of Filtered Waste Products
from Kidneys to Urethra.

from other conditions such as lupus (an immune system disorder), AIDS, hepatitis B, or hepatitis C, these are not the most frequent culprits. The most common causes are—take a guess—diabetes and high blood pressure. This news is especially distressing for African Americans, who suffer from these illnesses in greater numbers than the general population. In addition, research is beginning to suggest a possible genetic predisposition towards end-stage renal disease in African Americans. The discussions below examine some of the causes of kidney disease.

Diabetes

As explained in Chapter 4, diabetes causes your blood sugar levels—that is, the amount of glucose in your blood—to rise. Over time, high blood sugar levels can damage the blood vessels that serve your kidneys and enable them to filter waste products out of the blood. This can cause inflammation in those vessels, initiating a chain reaction of bad consequences. By damaging the circulatory system, diabetes can also have a destructive effect on the nerves in your body—which, like other parts of your body, are served by the blood vessels. In addition to causing other problems, damage to the nerves makes it difficult for you to empty your bladder. This, in turn, creates infections in the urinary tract that can back up into your kidneys, causing more damage.

Hypertension

Chapter 3 describes how hypertension forces the heart to work harder, which damages blood vessels throughout the body, including those found in the kidneys. Over time, the gradual increase in blood pressure takes its toll on the kidneys, adversely affecting their blood flow and those special filtering tubules. This sets up a vicious circle of events. As the kidneys incur damage, they become less able to perform their necessary functions, including waste (urine) removal, the regulation of the body's water levels, and the production of renin, which helps control blood pressure. Of course, this simply creates a further elevation in blood pressure, which means more damage to the kidneys, and so on. An estimated

25,000 new cases of kidney failure are caused by hypertension in the United States every year.

Sadly, in the projects where I grew up, most people never thought that they might have high blood pressure, and I suspect that many still don't. I believe that most also don't realize that there's a cause-and-effect relationship between hypertension and kidney disease. This is unfortunate, as the occurrence of hypertension—which is caused not only by diet but also by high levels of socioeconomic stress—is higher in the Black population and especially in the projects.

Drugs and Toxins

The prolonged overuse of painkillers such as acetaminophen (Tylenol), ibuprofen (Advil), and naproxen (Aleve) may result in injury to the kidneys through a process called *analgesic nephropathy*, another cause of kidney disease. The use of illegal intravenous drugs has also been connected to renal failure. Finally, kidney disease has been associated with environmental factors such as heavy metals, industrial chemicals, and viral infections.

Genetics

The rate of death from heart disease is 50 percent higher for Black Americans than it is for White Americans, while the death rate from stroke is 80 percent higher for Black Americans than it is for White Americans. These statistics, however, don't even come close to the prevalence of kidney failure in the Black community. The rate of end-stage renal disease is an incredible 320 percent higher for Black Americans than it is for White Americans. Although kidney disease is associated with other health conditions common to the Black community, such as high blood pressure and diabetes, not to mention socioeconomic factors, these reasons alone do not account for the overwhelming prevalence of the illness in African Americans. In fact, some of the most interesting research suggests a genetic predisposition to the problem.

Combine this potential genetic predisposition to kidney disease with the occurrence of hypertension, diabetes, and socioeconomic stress, and you have a formula that explains the staggering death rate from end-stage renal disease in the Black community.

Obesity

It has already been pointed out repeatedly in this book that obesity plays a significant role in the development of type 2 diabetes and hypertension, both of which are major contributors to kidney failure. What you may not know is that obesity has been linked to end-stage renal disease independent of diabetes and high blood pressure. The heavier you are, the more work your kidneys have to do to keep your body functioning properly. Eventually, these organs can simply get worn out and fail.

HOW DO YOU REDUCE THE RISK OF KIDNEY DISEASE?

Although kidney disease may seem inevitable, the remarkable truth is that it is highly preventable—even for African Americans, who may have a genetic predisposition to kidney failure. Even in the case of a genetic predisposition, it is far from true that the outcome is already determined. Why? Genetic predisposition often requires the right environment and circumstances in order for the predisposition to spur development of the disease. If the right circumstances are not present, there's a good chance that the disease will not occur.

By taking steps to control or avoid the conditions that contribute to a decline in renal function, you can overcome these potential problems. This means that you must control your blood pressure and blood sugar by using many of the same methods mentioned in other chapters. The following recommendations are not only ways to prevent or treat kidney disease but also ways to improve your overall health, which will have a protective effect against a number of illnesses.

Exercise

There is simply no substitute for physical activity when it comes to benefiting your long-term health. Exercise helps maintain proper blood sugar levels, alleviates high blood pressure, and fights obesity. In doing so, it reduces the burden placed on the kidneys. Exercise also helps decrease stress, thereby eliminating the damaging compounds produced by this condition. Thirty minutes of moderate physical activity a day—even if that activity merely consists of going for a walk—will do you a world of good. (To learn more about exercise, see page 41.)

Lose Weight

Losing weight is one of the best things you can do for your health. Shedding those extra pounds will improve kidney function by lightening the workload they are forced to bear every day. Of course, slimming down will also help you alleviate or even avoid type 2 diabetes and high blood pressure, which constitute the two biggest causative factors of kidney disease. For example, research has shown that blood pressure begins to decline with a 10-percent loss of total body weight. Because a healthful body weight is good for your system in so many ways, its importance should not be underestimated or ignored. (For information on losing weight, see page 38 in Chapter 2.)

Reduce Stress

Stress causes your system to secrete a rush of hormones, such as cortisol and norepinephrine. These hormones raise your blood pressure, preparing you to either fight the stressor or flee from it. Although it is only a temporary reaction, the elevation in blood pressure can still damage blood vessels, which can lead to impaired kidney function. Also, as explained in the inset found on page 19 of Chapter 1, in the twenty-first century, stress is ongoing and often leads to chronic increases in blood pressure and blood glucose.

While you may know about the importance of reducing your stress level, it is easier said than done. Steps you can take to decrease stress include exercise, breathing slowly, getting proper rest, meditation, prayer, and simplifying your life.

You may also consider taking a supplement called L-theanine, an amino acid that has been shown to reduce mental and physical stress while improving your cognition and mood. It does so by increasing the level of a neurotransmitter called gamma-aminobutyric acid, which regulates your brain's response; and dopamine, a brain-calming and signaling chemical that enhances cognition. Doses can range from 50 mg to 200 mg daily, with a maximum recommended daily amount of 1,200 mg.

First mentioned in Chapter 4, DHEA, or dehydroepiandrosterone, is a naturally occurring hormone that is produced by the adrenal glands. In Chapter 4, DHEA was suggested to improve insulin sensitivity, but it also balances your fight-or-flight response. As a result, this supplement is helpful during times of stress. I suggest that women take 25 mg per day and men take 50 mg per day.

Reduce Your Salt Intake

People with reduced kidney function also have an impaired ability to excrete salt. Excess salt in the body causes water retention, which increases blood pressure, and increased blood pressure further damages the kidneys, limiting their ability to rid the body of salt. In this case, a low-salt diet is advised.

The recommended daily intake of salt for healthy individuals is 2,400 mg, or about 1 teaspoon—although the average American consumes far more than this amount, A low-salt diet would supply between 1,000 mg and 2,000 mg daily, depending on your condition. Using salt substitutes is another option, but if you already have kidney disease, you'll want to steer clear of substitutes that are high in potassium. An easy method to monitor the amount of salt in your diet is to salt your food only after it has been prepared and not during cooking. That way, you can use as little as you please. Another option is to avoid added salt entirely and learn to use salt-free spices and herbs to flavor your foods. And don't forget to check the Nutrition Facts labels on any processed foods you buy. Even if you don't add further salt, many processed products already include more salt than you should have.

Finally, consider following the DASH Diet, which was designed to lower high blood pressure. It involves eating a diet rich in whole grains, fruits, vegetables, and low-fat dairy products, as well as some fish, poultry, and legumes. For more information about the DASH Diet, see page 169 of Chapter 9 and check page 286 of the Resources section. It is important to note that if you already suffer from renal disease, you must work with a dietician to develop a food plan that's right for your specific needs. Other nutrients—such as phosphorous, potassium, calcium, and protein—may also have to be limited.

Take Vitamin D$_3$

As you learned in Chapter 3 on hypertension, vitamin D$_3$ has demonstrated the ability to lower blood pressure by preventing the overproduction of the hormone renin. In this manner, vitamin D$_3$ has a protective effect on the kidneys, fending off damage that can lead to or worsen kidney disease. In addition to this benefit, vitamin D$_3$ hinders the development of fibrosis, the formation of internal scar tissue that can cause devastating effects in the kidneys. Finally, vitamin D$_3$ helps counteract the anemia that often results from chronic kidney disease.

I recommend taking between 2,000 and 5,000 IU of vitamin D$_3$ per day as a protective measure, depending on your current blood levels of the nutrient. Before starting supplementation, it's a good idea to ask your physician to order a blood test that will check your current vitamin D$_3$ levels. Make sure that your physician orders the 25-OH vitamin D test, which is the most accurate method available today.

Take Vitamin K$_2$

Vitamin K$_2$ can help you avoid the typical hardening of the arteries associated with kidney disease. It supports proper calcium metabolism, preventing calcium from being deposited in inappropriate places in your body, including your blood vessels. The recommended daily allowance of this nutrient is 80 mcg for men and 65 mcg for women. While it is possible to get your daily dose of vitamin K$_2$ from dietary sources such as leafy greens and vegetables, most people would benefit from supplementation.

Consider Traditional Medication

Depending on your health status and the effectiveness of the life-style changes and supplements discussed in this chapter, you may have to rely on traditional medication to prevent or treat kidney disease.

Kidney disease patients are usually given a *diuretic*, also called a water pill, as a first line of defense. Most commonly prescribed in the form of hydrochlorothiazide, a mild diuretic is one of the oldest means of inhibiting water retention and controlling blood pressure in cases of kidney disease and hypertension. Should this single medication not work, you may be asked to take an *ACE inhibitor* (angiotensin-converting enzyme inhibitor) or an *ARB blocker* (angiotensin receptor blocker) as well. ACE inhibitors reduce kidney damage by dilating blood vessels, while ARB blockers have a similar effect by preventing blood vessels from narrowing.

Other medications that alleviate high blood pressure and thus slow the destruction of the kidneys include *beta-blockers*, which decrease heart rate; *calcium channel blockers*, which relax muscles in the walls of blood vessels; and *vasodilators*, which also relax blood vessel walls. However, just being on a drug doesn't mean that everything is under control. It isn't. If you are given a medication, ask your provider how the medication will help you and enquire about its side effects. The more you know, the more control you will have over your situation.

Ultimately, any medication has its pros and cons, all of which should be discussed with your provider so that you can make an informed decision about your treatment. If you are working with a doctor because you already have kidney disease, be sure to consult him before adding any supplements to your regimen.

CONCLUSION

The evidence is clear. Hypertension and diabetes are the two biggest risk factors for kidney disease—and more than likely are preceded by weight issues. Neglecting to treat these disorders with every method at your disposal can be disastrous to your well-being. Once it takes hold, kidney disease affects your quality of life in every way imaginable. It has dire financial and emotional costs and wide-ranging effects on your health. These facts are especially alarming for African Americans, not only because they are more likely to suffer from hypertension and diabetes, but also because they are more likely to see these illnesses lead to fatal end-stage kidney disease. But do not despair. While statistics and even the recognition of a possible genetic predisposition should raise your awareness of the problem, they should not extinguish hope. You can prevent renal disease, and if you have it, you can take steps to better manage it.

Your first line of defense is your knowledge of the lifestyle choices you can make to improve your health. These should include watching your weight, maintaining a healthful diet (cutting down on salt, in particular), exercising, and reducing your levels of stress. Each of these lifestyle choices works against the damaging effects of high blood pressure and diabetes, thus helping you avoid the destruction of your kidneys. In addition, incorporating a vitamin D_3 supplement into your health regimen is one of the best and easiest things you can do to fight renal failure. In fact, vitamin D_3 can help lower the risk of kidney failure associated with hypertension and type 2 diabetes and also appears to lessen some of the harmful symptoms of kidney disease, should you already be affected by the illness. Other common supplements, such as DHEA, can also help you maintain kidney health.

Finally, traditional medication is available and should not be discounted. Lifestyle adjustments and nutritional supplements are powerful tools against kidney disease, but a doctor's prescription is never to be ignored. Always speak to your healthcare provider about all forms of treatment so that you can take full advantage of the options available to you.

7

Cancer

*"The ultimate measure of a man is not where he stands
in moments of comfort and convenience, but where
he stands at a time of challenge and controversy."*
—DR. MARTIN LUTHER KING, JR.

The good news is this: Since 1990, the overall cancer death rate has dropped faster in Blacks than Whites among both men and women, largely driven by more rapid declines in Blacks for lung, colorectal, and prostate cancer. The bad news—and it is bad—is that African Americans with cancer still have the highest death rates and shortest survival rates of any racial and ethnic group in the United States. Compared with White males, African-American males are more likely to be diagnosed with lung, prostate, and stomach cancer, and have lower five-year survival rates from lung and pancreatic cancer. Although African-American women are slightly less likely than their White counterparts to be diagnosed with breast cancer, they are much more likely to die of it. Their chance of acquiring stomach cancer is double that of White women, and they are twice as likely to succumb to the disease.

The fact that African-American deaths from cancer are greater than those of Whites should come as no surprise. Based on all the factors that are working against us, it's a wonder we don't have even higher cancer and death rates. The reality is that without making an effort to protect ourselves, we are sitting ducks—and the conditions that underlie cancer are unlikely to go away.

Fortunately, there are things you can do today to protect yourself and your loved ones from this terrible disease.

It would be nice if I could give a complete and simple explanation for African-American cancer statistics and then give you a simple plan for changing these alarming numbers. Unfortunately, I cannot. When dealing with cancer, answers are often complex and hard to come by. But let us not discount the fact that there *are* some answers. One way in which you can help avoid cancer, for instance, is to take a daily dose of a vitamin your body requires. There is considerable evidence that vitamin D3 deficiency contributes to the formation and proliferation of cancer cells, which suggests that an increase in vitamin D3 intake in the Black community (or any community) could potentially curb its staggering cancer rates. This information is vital to initiating a positive change in the health of African Americans, not to mention the country as a whole.

It's always best to begin at the beginning, so this chapter starts by explaining what cancer is. We then discuss the many causes of cancer, from environmental toxins to diet. Finally, and most important, we discuss the ways in which you can reduce your risk of this insidious disease.

Remember that statistics and research data are always changing. These dire cancer predictions are not set in stone and are not the ultimate determinants of the future of Black America. We *can* change the facts, so let us begin to do so by learning about cancer.

WHAT IS CANCER?

From the moment you begin to develop in the womb, all of your body's cells are programmed to duplicate in a fixed manner to allow you to grow and mature. In the same way, when you have a skin injury such as a cut, your skin cells duplicate just enough to heal the injury, and they then stop growing.

Sometimes, though, cells lose their ability to duplicate normally. Whether caused by random error, inherited abnormality, or environmental factors called *carcinogens*, the genetic information, or DNA, of a cell can be damaged, and that damage can produce mutations in the cell. If the mutated cell begins to reproduce itself without restriction, those abnormal cells often form a mass—a tumor. This process of uncontrolled cell division can arise from any type of cell, in any organ, including the blood.

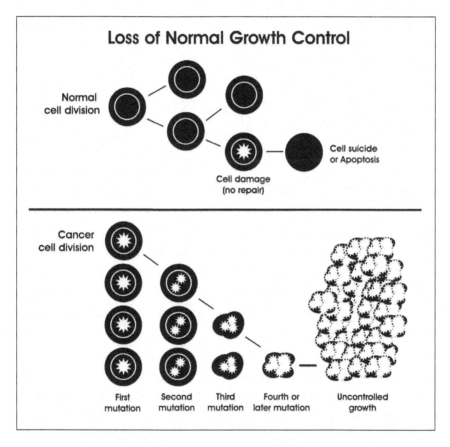

Figure 7.1. Normal versus Abnormal Cell Division.

Figure 7.1 illustrates two types of cell division. The top example shows a mutated cell undergoing cellular suicide. Thankfully, one of the miracles of human life is that every cell in the body is preprogrammed to self-destruct once it recognizes that something is wrong with its development. This process is called *apoptosis* and is initiated by the p53 gene, also known as the tumor-suppressing gene. If this gene is turned off because of damage or genetic abnormality, however, it will not allow the abnormal cell to recognize its own mutation. As depicted in the bottom example of the figure, the abnormal cell will continue to survive and multiply, forming a tumor.

The formation of a tumor, however, does not necessarily mean cancer. All tumors are not cancerous, although the words *tumor* and *cancer* are often used synonymously. When discussing tumors, the two most important terms to understand are malignant and benign. If a tumor is *benign*, it is not cancerous. This kind of tumor generally has a limit to its growth and does not spread. Just as important, most of the time, it does not return once it has been removed. One example of a common benign tumor is uterine fibroids, which are small growths in the uterus.

Malignant tumors, on the other hand, are cancerous. They have the potential to invade other tissues and spread throughout the body through a process called *metastasis*. While most cancers are marked by the presence of a tumor, some, such as leukemia, are not.

WHAT CAUSES CANCER?

The potential for cancer exists in your body as long as its cells are thriving and dividing, which is basically as long as you are alive. Imperfect cells that can cause cancer usually arise because of damage from free radicals, which are generated inside the body. (See the inset on free radicals on page 47 of Chapter 2.) These unstable molecules are truly destructive and have been linked to many diseases. While they can be created by exposure to factors such as cigarette smoke and asbestos, they also spring up unavoidably through the natural functions of the body. Free radicals can sometimes injure the previously mentioned p53 gene, turning it off and thereby allowing cancers to flourish.

That being said, there are many lifestyle choices, substances in the environment, and other factors that have been shown to contribute to the development of cancer. Below, you'll learn about the most common of these contributing causes.

Alcohol

Right now, you may be thinking, "Alcohol, really?" If you have been unaware until now of the link between alcohol and cancer, you are not alone. Seven out of ten American have never heard of alcohol's connection to cancer. Consuming any type of alcohol raises your risk of acquiring a variety of cancers, including cancer of the mouth, throat, larynx (voice box), esophagus (food pipe), liver, breast, colon, and rectum. The more you drink, the greater your risk of getting one of these cancers.

Cigarettes

While smoking cigarettes is also associated with heart and lung disease and stroke, there is no question that it is linked to many types of cancer. Cigarette smoke contains hundreds of harmful chemicals, dozens of which have been officially classified as carcinogens. These chemicals include arsenic, benzene, cadmium, nickel, ethylene oxide, and beryllium, to name just a few. In addition to being a leading cause of lung cancer, cigarette smoke has been linked to cancers of the larynx, oral cavity and pharynx, esophagus, pancreas, bladder, stomach, colon and rectum, liver, cervix, and kidneys, as well as to acute myeloid leukemia, a cancer of the blood and bone marrow. It's important to note that as second-hand smoke is inhaled by a smoker's family members, their odds of getting one of these cancers also increases.

Diet

There are a number of dietary factors that can influence your chance of getting cancer. A diet that is high in fat has consistently been associated with an increased risk of numerous forms of cancer, as well as with obesity, which is itself a cancer risk because it alters the bacteria that make up the microbiome. (See Chapter 1 to learn about the microbiome and Chapter 2 to learn about obesity.) Low-fiber diets have also been associated with an increased risk of cancer. And to a lesser degree, cancer has been linked to high red meat intake, especially when the meat is cooked at high temperatures, releasing chemicals that can damage your cells. (See the inset below.)

Further, processed foods appear to contribute to cancer beyond their tendency to lead to weight gain. According to an unpublished internal study of the FDA, the food products produced by US food processing plants contain high levels of heavy metals, chlorine, pesticides, and other toxic chemicals that are known carcinogens. Unfortunately, without the proper monitoring, that leaves a good deal of the processed foods found on our supermarket shelves questionable in regard to their effect on cancer risk.

Environmental Toxins

Environmental toxins are chemicals and other environmental factors—both manmade and naturally occurring—that can harm your

---

WHAT'S IN YOUR WELL-DONE HAMBURGER?

It may taste good and look great, especially when you're enjoying yourself at a summer barbecue, but there is more inside that char-grilled burger than you know. Here are a few chemicals that are likely to be present in a well-done beef patty:

- heterocyclic amines [e.g. 2-amino-1-methyl1–6-phenyl-imidazo[4,5-b]pyridine (PhIP);

- 2-amino-3,8-dimethylimidazo-[4,5-b]quinoxaline (MelQx);

- 2-amino-3, 4,8-trimethylimidazo-[4,5-f]quinoxaline (DiMelQx); and

- polycyclic aromatic hydrocarbons [e.g. benzo(a)pyrene (BaP)]." (16, 17)

As mentioned on page 125, beef cooked at high heat produces chemicals that have been shown to increase your risk of cancer. So while you may not choose to entirely avoid these treats, you should consider eating them only on an occasional basis.

health by disrupting sensitive biological systems. We now know that many environmental toxins can lead to cancer.

Unfortunately, environmental toxics can be found almost everywhere. From the gases given off during the manufacturing of chemicals to the waste products dumped into the rivers and streams by thousands of manufacturers—from the old lead paints found on walls to the lead pipes carrying our water supplies—we are surrounded by these potentially carcinogenic substances. Many of these chemicals can damage our genetic material either individually or when they are combined with other chemicals. And since our bodies have no natural way of eliminating these toxins, they build up in our cells over time. The consequences are even worse if we are overweight or obese, because these toxins are stored in fat cells.

Below, we'll focus on two environmental toxins that have especially strong links to cancer.

Asbestos

Asbestos is a fibrous material composed of six naturally occurring silicate minerals. Due to its physical properties, before it was recognized as a cancer-causing substance, asbestos was used as insulation in schools, factories, and homes; as insulation, a fireproofing material, and a building material in ships; and in the manufacture of automobile parts, textiles, and even talcum powder. Shipbuilders during World War II as well as workers in factories that produced asbestos-containing products were particularly exposed to large amounts of asbestos dust, which remains in the lungs once breathed in.

Exposure to asbestos can cause cancers of the lung, larynx, and ovary, but *mesothelioma*—a cancer of the thin membranes that line the chest and abdomen—is the most common form of cancer associated with exposure to asbestos. Although its use is not as widespread as it once was, asbestos may still be present in old homes and workplaces.

Radiation

Radiation is essentially waves of energy that exist at different frequencies. High frequency radiation negatively affects your body by removing electrons from the atoms in your body, thereby creating free radicals, which can damage your DNA and ultimately result in cancer. This process is called *ionization*. Sources of ionizing radiation include cosmic rays, natural radiation from the earth, medical diagnostic tests, nuclear weapons, and, to a degree, ultraviolet light. While non-ionizing sources of radiation such as power lines, televisions, and cell phones have been called into question as possible carcinogens, no concrete link has been made between them and cancer.

Genetic Predisposition

An inherited mutation of certain tumor-suppressing genes has been linked to the increased likelihood of an individual getting cancer. In addition, some scientists argue for the presence of a cancer-causing gene, also called an *oncogene*, which may be more likely to be activated in certain people than in others. But much more research must be done, and it is important to remember that having a predisposition to cancer is not a guarantee that you will acquire the disease. However, if one of your grandparents, parents, or siblings had a specific type of cancer, you should make sure that you are tested to rule out that you have it. Testing is particularly important for those with a family history of breast or ovarian cancers.

Genetic tests are available for some types of cancer, including the following: breast, colon, connective tissue (sarcoma), kidney, ovarian, pancreatic, prostate, skin (melanoma), and stomach. Speak to your healthcare provider or contact the American Cancer Society about these tests. Also speak to your healthcare provider about the diagnostic tests that can alert you to the presence of cancer at early stages, when it is most treatable. These are discussed on page 136 of this chapter.

Viruses

Although it is rare to acquire cancer from a virus, there are a handful of viruses that have been linked to certain forms of the disease, such as the human T-cell lymphotrophic virus (HTLV), which can lead to adult T-cell leukemia, and the human papillomavirus (HPV), which can lead to cervical cancer. The association between cervical cancer and the human papillomavirus is so strong, in fact, that the medical community recommends HPV vaccination for girls and boys as early as age nine to protect them from HPV infections that can cause cancer later in their lives. The vaccine has been proven to be most effective if provided before the individual has any sexual contact.

Vitamin D₃ Deficiency

As you'll learn throughout this book, low levels of vitamin D_3 can contribute to a number of health issues, including a weakened immune system, infections, colds, fatigue, body aches, depression, bone loss, hair loss, and diabetes. However, after evaluating the data related to cancer in the Black population, I believe that low vitamin D_3 levels also contribute to the development of cancer.

In the Vitamin D and Omega-3 Trial (VITAL), published in 2020, researchers studied the independent effects of vitamin D and omega-3 fatty acid supplementation on the risk for developing cancer. Some subjects received only placebos, some received a placebo for one supplement but not the other, and some received both supplements. The trial was performed using both White and Black subjects. Although in their final report, the researchers concluded that there was no clear-cut decrease in the incidence of cancers in those taking vitamin D, an examination of the data actually shows a 23-percent decrease in the occurrence of cancer in African-American participants who took this supplement.

Why, despite the results experienced by African-American participants, did researchers conclude that there was no relationship between vitamin D_3 intake and lower cancer rates? Did the researchers simply discount the significance of the vitamin to Black Americans? While the misleading study conclusion is disturbing, the bottom line is that low vitamin D_3 levels in Blacks may be an unrecognized cause of many cancers in our communities—and it is time we sound the alarm.

HOW CAN YOU REDUCE THE RISK OF CANCER?

Our knowledge of cancer—what it is and what causes it—shows us that we can play an important part in lowering cancer risk. We can make important lifestyle changes, we can take supplements that have been shown to be beneficial, and we can make sure to get the physical examinations and tests that can alert us to cancer in early stages, when the disease is most treatable.

Make Healthy Lifestyle Changes

It's hard to change old habits. Some of them may have come about because everyone around you shares these same habits. Some of them may be a reaction to the stress of your daily life. Regardless of why you adopted them, they are now part of how you live each day, and modifying them is far from easy. However, if these practices have been shown to increase your risk of getting cancer, perhaps it's time for a change. The following actions can help save your life.

Quit Smoking

Smoking is one of the most harmful things you can do to your body, and the link between cigarettes and numerous types of cancer has been solidly established. It seems like every year, research shows a connection between this nasty habit and yet another form of the disease. In fact, quitting smoking is probably the single most important thing you could do to lower your cancer risk. (It will also help you avoid heart disease, which is no small thing.)

If you are a smoker, please do not wait another day to stop. I know that it's a tough addiction to break, but millions of people have done it. If you don't want to do it for yourself, do it for the people who love you. And if you find that you can't quit smoking without help—and many people can't—speak to your doctor about patches, gums, and other aids that can assist you in making this important change.

Limit Your Alcohol Consumption

Sometimes you just need a drink to relax, right? Maybe your parents drink, your siblings drink, and your friends drink, so why not you? As discussed earlier in this chapter, drinking alcohol increases your odds of getting cancer. I am not telling you to stop drinking alcohol completely, but the less you drink, the lower your chances of getting any type of cancer. One glass of wine, okay. Half a bottle, not so much. One beer, okay. A full six pack, no.

Change Your Diet

Research suggests that lowering the amount of fat in your diet also lowers your risk of contracting colon, prostate, and breast cancer. Studies also show an association between diets that are high in fiber and decreased rates of stomach and colorectal cancer. In addition, populations that consume lots of fruits, vegetables, and whole grains consistently display lower rates of numerous forms of cancer than those that do not. Finally, there is evidence that the higher a population's intake of animal protein, the higher its rates of numerous cancers.

In earlier chapters, I've recommended food plans such as the Mediterranean Diet, which includes healthy amounts of vegetables, fruits, and grains and limited amounts of lean protein. A diet such as this can help you minimize your risk of cancer and a number of other serious disorders. (For more information about healthful diets, see page 166 of Chapter 9.)

Get More Sunshine

Most people get their vitamin D from food and sunshine. As discussed elsewhere in this book, obtaining an adequate amount of this vitamin from foods is not easy because most of us don't consume sufficient amounts of the few foods that contain significant amounts of vitamin D—fatty fish, such as salmon, mackerel, and sardines; cod liver oil; beef liver; and egg yolks. This why it's so important to spend more time out in the sun. You see, when your skin is exposed to sunlight, it makes vitamin D from cholesterol.

Understanding the Relationship between Vitamin D₃ and Cancer

The mechanism through which vitamin D_3 decreases the risk of cancer is complex and beyond the scope of this book. However, there are some concepts you should understand. Vitamin D_3 is *not* an antioxidant that scavenges free radicals. Rather, it protects genes and cells in a very different way.

Recent cancer research tells us that when cells are in contact with one another, both their signaling between each other and their protection of one another are improved. This contact may also increase the effectiveness of *apoptosis*, the normal programmed cell death that is lacking in cancer.

A deficiency in vitamin D_3 decreases the adhesiveness of cells, allowing them to lose contact with one another. When this occurs, cells begin to function independently, leading to a host of adverse actions that may result in uncontrolled tumor growth. At every step of this abnormal process, restoration of adequate levels of vitamin D_3 can help return normal cellular function. In some cases, vitamin D acts to stimulate the production of certain proteins, and in other cases, it affects gene behavior by attaching to genetic material like the vitamin D receptor (VDR) site located in DNA material.

Although vitamin D clearly plays a significant role in normal cell function and helps guard against the development of cancer, it's important to note that this supplement is not all powerful. Even if there are adequate amounts of vitamin D_3 present in the body, high amounts of offending agents—such as tobacco smoke (nicotine); mycotoxins (the toxic material produced by mold); toxic chemicals such as benzene; or dietary fats—can overwhelm the vitamin's protective benefits. The bottom line is that in addition to getting adequate D_3, it is vital to avoid lifestyle habits and toxins that increase the risk of cancer.

The sun's ultraviolet B (UVB) rays hit cholesterol in the skin cells, providing the energy for vitamin D synthesis to occur.

How much sun exposure do you need to get the vitamin D your body requires? Because the high amount of melanin in African-American skin blocks many of the UVB rays, you should aim for ninety minutes of sunlight three times a week. Ideally, you should bare your face, arms, and trunk; use no sunscreen; and plan to be out in the midday sun, which is the strongest.

If you are thinking that getting this much sun would be a difficult task, you're not alone. Especially if you live in an area that is cold in the winter, it may be impossible to get all the sun you need. My recommendation is that you increase your sun exposure as much as possible and also take vitamin D supplements, which are discussed on page 136.

Take Supplements

Research has shown that some supplements can improve your body's ability to prevent the occurrence of cancer and, in some cases, may even help your body fight the disease. The supplements listed below have all been found beneficial. For guidance in choosing the best-quality supplements and using them effectively, see the inset on page 134. For a more complete guide to anti-cancer supplements, see page 263.

Curcumin (Turmeric)

Turmeric is a spice commonly used in Indian curries, where it provides both a distinctive flavor and a rich color. Its most biologically active component, curcumin, is also known for its potential anti-cancer activity. One of the most amazing things about curcumin is that it seems to stop the progression of cancer cells without affecting healthy cells.

While more research is required to determine the optimal amount needed, 50 to 100 mg per day is considered an appropriate dose of pure curcumin extract, although people have been known to take higher doses. The most typical side effects of high dosages include nausea and diarrhea. Curcumin should not be taken by individuals undergoing chemotherapy, as it may make the treatment less effective.

Omega-3 Fatty Acids

Omega-3 fatty acids are necessary to maintain good health but cannot be manufactured by the body. They must be obtained through diet—usually through the consumption of fatty fish, such as salmon—or through supplementation. Although more research is needed, some studies have shown that adults who maintain an omega-3 fatty acid intake of 1 to 3 grams per day are less likely to develop cancer of the colon, breast, and prostate.

Probiotics

Also referred to as "friendly bacteria," probiotics—first discussed

---

CHOOSING THE BEST SUPPLEMENTS

As we discuss throughout this book, nutritional supplements can be beneficial in maintaining normal body function and defending against serious disorders. However, not all supplements are equal. Some do not contain the nutrient promised on the label, and some are not well absorbed by the body. That's why it makes sense to know a little about supplements before spending your hard-earned money on them.

To be sure you are truly getting what the supplement says it contains, visit the website ConsumerLab.com. This nonprofit independent organization tests different brands of many different supplements and then determines which ones contain what their labels say they contain and also offer the best price. It costs a few dollars a month to access the information on this website, but in the end, the information may actually save you money by guiding you to the best brands.

When purchasing supplements, the best choice is a pharmaceutical-grade product. In order to be certified pharmaceutical grade, the supplement must exceed 99-percent purity and not in Chapter 1—are microorganisms that live in the digestive tract and perform a variety of helpful functions. By inhibiting the proliferation of potentially cancer-promoting bacteria, neutralizing other carcinogenic agents, and boosting the immune system, probiotics are thought to be especially protective against colon cancer.

You can get friendly bacteria by eating probiotic foods such as yogurt or by taking probiotic supplements. If you opt for supplements, I recommend choosing a product that provides at least five different types of bacteria and more than 70 billion colonies per dose. (For more information on probiotic foods and supplements, see page 22.) If you are undergoing chemotherapy, talk to your doctor before taking probiotic supplements.

contain any fillers, binders, or other inactive ingredients. These supplements are also highly bioavailable, meaning that your body can more easily absorb and use the nutrients they provide. If you're buying supplements in the store, ask the salesperson to guide you to pharmaceutical-grade brands. If ordering online, check the website or contact the company to get information on the supplement's grade. Be aware that only a small percentage of the supplements on the market are of pharmaceutical grade, so you may have to do some hunting to find them. If you can't locate pharmaceutical-grade supplements, buy whole food-based supplements, which are sourced from actual food and contain natural compounds that increase bioavailability.

Before you purchase a supplement, make sure that it's the specific form recommended in this book—for instance, be certain you have vitamin D_3 and not vitamin D_2—and check the dosage so that you'll be able to easily take the recommended amount. To increase absorbability, unless otherwise directed, take supplements with a meal rather than on an empty stomach. For more information on buying and using supplements, see the Guide to Dietary Supplements section that begins on page 258.

Vitamin D$_3$

As you learned in earlier chapters, getting enough vitamin D is important for preventing many illnesses. And as shown in the VITAL study, discussed on page 129, the use of vitamin D supplements may decrease the occurrence of cancer in African Americans by as much as 23 percent. Research has shown that vitamin D may slow tumor growth, inhibit the spread of cancer, have anti-inflammatory effects, promote cell death, and decrease tumor invasiveness.

Because of the high amount of the pigment melanin in the skin of African Americans, it is difficult for our bodies to synthesize adequate amounts of vitamin D from exposure to sun. Moreover, both Black and White people usually don't get the vitamin D they need from foods. Therefore, if you are at high risk for getting cancer or are already fighting cancer, I recommend that you take at least 5,000 IU of vitamin D$_3$ per day. You can also ask your healthcare provider to test your vitamin D levels and prescribe a dosage based on the results. Make sure that your physician orders the 25-OH vitamin D test, as this will give you the best indication of your current vitamin D body stores.

Vitamin K$_2$

While researching bone loss in women with cirrhosis of the liver, Japanese scientists stumbled across data suggesting that vitamin K$_2$ may offer protection against cancer. To their surprise, women who had been given vitamin K$_2$ supplements were 90 percent less likely to develop liver cancer, a common result of cirrhosis of the liver, than those who had not. Moreover, a German study proved a link between increased levels of vitamin K$_2$ and a decrease in prostate cancer in men.

The recommended daily allowance of vitamin K$_2$ is 70 to 80 mcg per day for men, and 55 to 65 mcg per day for women.

Get Diagnostic Tests

Unfortunately, too few of us in the Black community go to a doctor when we should and get the standard tests that are available to safeguard our health. It may be a lack of access, or it may be because of the costs involved. Some people just learn to live with the pain or other symptoms—until they can't.

Earlier, on page 128, you learned that genetic testing can alert you to a predisposition to some forms of cancer. Just as important, the following tests can alert you to cancer—often at an early stage—so that you can begin treatment as soon as possible. Discuss these tests with your healthcare provider so that you have the best possible chance of detecting and successfully managing cancer.

COMPLETE BLOOD COUNT (CBC). Besides telling you a great deal about your general health, the CBC can signal some forms of cancer. High numbers of white blood cells—associated with fatigue, bruising for seemingly no reason, nose bleeds, etc.—may indicate leukemia or lymphoma, two blood cancers, If you have too few red blood cells, sometimes referred to as a low hematocrit, there may be bleeding somewhere in your body, which could be a sign of cancer. This test should be performed every year.

BREAST EXAM. Another helpful diagnostic text is the breast exam—a simple physical exam provided by your healthcare provider to find lumps, which could be either cancerous or benign. Although routine breast self-exams used to be recommended, they are no longer advised simply because they have not been shown to be effective in detecting cancer. However, if you do detect a lump or other irregularity while taking a shower, for instance, you should immediately contact your healthcare provider.

MAMMOGRAM. An X-ray picture of the breast, this important test helps detect breast cancer. Women ages forty-five to fifty-four should get a mammogram every year. Women age fifty-five and older can switch to every two years or continue an annual exam.

Other tests, such as a thermography or an MRI, can also be used to detect breast cancer. However, the former is no longer recommended, and the latter is not as effective at early detection as a mammogram. The newer 3D mammogram, which combines multiple X-rays to create a three-dimensional picture of the breast, is proving effective in detecting breast cancer in women with dense breasts.

COLONOSCOPY. A colonoscopy can detect changes or abnormalities in the colon (large intestine) and rectum, including signs of cancer. During a colonoscopy, a long, flexible tube in inserted in the rectum and snaked through the large intestine, and a video camera at the tip of the tube allows the doctor to view the inside. If polyps (clump of cells growing on the inside wall of the intestine) are found, they are removed and sent to a laboratory to determine whether they are malignant or benign. Since a benign polyp can become cancerous, its removal may prevent future cancer.

An initial exam should be performed at age fifty. Exams should then be done every five or ten years. If you have a family history of colon cancer, your doctor may want to begin testing you at age forty.

If you do not have a family history of colon cancer and a previous colonoscopy has not shown polyps, your doctor may recommend that you use *Cologuard,* a home test that can detect problems through a stool sample. Be aware, though, that a Cologuard test is not as accurate as a colonoscopy, and of course, it does not include the removal of polyps.

DIGITAL RECTAL EXAM AND PSA TEST. In a digital rectal exam (DRE), the healthcare provider examines a man's lower rectum, pelvis, and lower belly to find evidence of prostate or rectal cancer or other problems. The doctor should also perform a testicular exam to detect lumps. Ask your provider to show you how you can do your own. This test should be performed every year once you reach the age of forty-five—especially if you have a family history of protate cancer.

Some doctors also perform a prostate-specific antigen (PSA) test—a blood test that can detect prostate cancer at any early stage. However, a PSA test can be misleading. Talk to your doctor to see if a PSA test is right for you.

PAP TEST. Also called a pap smear, the pap test was designed to test for cervical cancer in women and can also detect human papillomavirus (HPV), which causes cervical cancer. The healthcare provider collects cells from the cervix, the lower, narrow end of your uterus at the top of your vagina. Early detection and treatment, especially when the woman is found to have abnormal or precancerous cells (a condition known as cervical dysplasia), has an excellent cure rate. Screening should start at age twenty-one or when the individual becomes sexually active. If normal, it should be repeated every three years. Your doctor can tell you how often a pap test is advisable for you.

Testing for cancer has become easier and less costly. Ask you healthcare professional what tests *you* should have, given your family history and risk factors. Although some tests may cost more, they are a good deal less expensive than paying for long term advanced cancer treatment.

CONCLUSION

I hope that this chapter has given you a sense of optimism in the face of the African-American community's high rates of cancer. Although the statistics are disturbing, there is truly no reason that you cannot change them for the better. By increasing your vitamin D3 intake, improving your diet, breaking the cigarette habit, and making other important changes, you can avoid cancer or help insure that it's detected when it is most treatable.

TIMELINES
THE RED CROSS

1941 to 1942. In 1941, the Red Cross Blood Donor Program was established to obtain much-needed blood for wounded soldiers. Many Blacks responded by attempting to donate blood, but were rejected even though health experts knew scientifically that there was no difference between the blood of Whites and Blacks. The reason was purely racial discrimination. By 1942, the Red Cross accepted Black donors, but their blood, so called "Negro blood," was to be used for Black soldiers only. This policy remained in place until 1950, when the Red Cross stopped requiring the segregation of blood by race. However, it was not until the late 1960s and early 1970s that Southern states such as Arkansas and Louisiana finally stopped the segregation of the blood supply, ending another shameful chapter in American history.

What's particularly disgraceful about the treatment of "Negro blood" by the Red Cross is that it was a Black doctor, Dr. Charles R. Drew, a surgeon and medical researcher, who mastered, refined, and developed techniques for transfusions, blood storage, and blood banking during WW II. His success at revolutionizing blood banking led him to become Director of the Red Cross Blood Bank and Assistant Director of the National Research Council, responsible for blood collection for the United States Navy and Army. In 1942, he resigned in protest of the United States War Department's policy that African-American blood be separated from the blood of White Americans.

8

The Aging Process

*"Age is just a number. Life and aging are the greatest gifts
that we could possibly ever have."*
—CICELY TYSON

D o you have relatives who have lived a long time? Hopefully, they have also been reasonably healthy over the
years. The good news is that the life span of Blacks has
improved over the last fifty years. In 1970, the life expectation was
60 for Black men and 68.3 for Black women. Today, the average life
span is approximately 72 for Black men and 78 for Black women.
Whites live approximately three and a half years longer.

When we consider averages, we throw everyone into the mix.
To get to that total figure, we add the number of deaths among
young people, middle-aged people, and the elderly—those over
65—to come up with an average. However, when you consider
the fact that a much higher percentage of our people die of heart
attacks, cancer, diabetes, and the other degenerative diseases we
cover in this book, an interesting fact emerges. While a decent
number of our Black men and women may live longer than the
stats indicate, a good percentage may die much earlier based on
the current CDC numbers. In plain English, Aunt Corinne lived to
be 95, but her two children died at ages 61 and 63. So that family's
average life span was 73.

Because of the high number of deaths due to these various
health disorders, we should have a better understanding of what
we can do to increase our own life spans. Hopefully, you will get a

few ideas as you read this chapter. At the same time, don't forget that improving the quality of life is just as important as lengthening life span.

THE TIME FACTOR

As we get older, the natural process of aging affects every cell in our body. While our immune system used to respond quickly to an infection, inflammation, or virus when we were young, it slows down as we get older. Over the years, every cell in every organ experiences damage from environmental toxins that enter the body, poor nutrition that damages our cells, lack of exercise, or the natural effects of aging.

What this means is that the longer you live, the more damage your system undergoes. This makes your body less effective at fighting further damage, causing you to incur more damage, and so on. Fortunately, this doesn't mean that you can't substantially alter those processes that could accelerate aging and maintain your health for years to come. Watching what you eat, keeping your weight down, maintaining a proper vitamin intake, and carrying out a daily exercise routine are all ways in which you can lessen the effects of aging and stave off many of the diseases that have come to accompany growing older.

WHAT CONTRIBUTES TO AGING?

Medical researchers have studied why our bodies age—from why our organs deteriorate to why our hair turns gray and our skin wrinkles. And while they may have not discovered a treatment, their studies have uncovered some important information. By understanding the "why" of aging, we can better understand what we can do to slow it down. Much of the findings have to do with changes in the microbiome and the deterioration of cells, which is partly due to free radical damage.

Changes in Your Microbiome

Recent research has shown that the microbiome—the bacteria that live in your body—is strongly related to aging. As explained in

Chapter 1, a healthy microbiome, which provides diverse types of beneficial bacteria, is needed for a healthy immune system, to generate nutrition in human cells, and for so much more. Unfortunately, by the age of 60, your microbiome becomes less diverse, and the numbers of good bacteria have declined.

These alterations in the microbiome occur, at least in part, because the foods we eat often change as we age. Dental problems can cause chewing to be painful and difficult, making it harder to eat fruits, vegetable salads, and other nutrient- and fiber-packed foods. The process of cooking itself may change, because as muscles become weaker and movement becomes painful, it becomes more difficult to chop and otherwise prepare foods. Even moving around the kitchen from refrigerator to counter to stove can become harder. As a result, older people often eat a diet that includes too many sugary desserts, sweetened cereals, snack foods, white bread, peanut butter, potatoes, and pasta—foods that are cheap, easy to prepare, require little chewing, and taste good. However, all these foods are harmful to your microbiome. Damaging changes to the microbiome can also occur with the overuse of antibiotics, which kill good bacteria as well as bad.

When scientists studied the microbiome of older people and compared it with that of younger people, they noted an important change in the type of bacteria in the body. They saw a reduction in healthy bacteria and an increase in disease-promoting (opportunistic) bacteria—microbes that contribute to infection, cancer, and deficiencies in the immune system, all of which reduce life span.

Cell Deterioration

In general terms, the aging process is the natural deterioration of cellular function, and the truth is that no one really knows why cells degrade. This decline in cellular capability—called *senescence*—has significant effects on the human body.

To illustrate the biological transformations associated with aging, I will use the example of liver cells, also called *hepatocytes*. One of the most important operations of the liver is its role in detoxification of our blood. Unfortunately, as your liver ages, the effectiveness of the enzymes produced by the liver begins to decrease. Without properly functioning enzymes, the process of elimination of toxins begins to breaks down, and the toxins begin to accumulate throughout your body—in the cells, blood, tissues, brain, etc. The more toxins that remain in your body, the quicker the deterioration of the body's cells, because they interfere with normal metabolism. Thus begins a relentless process of degeneration. Cells grow old and lose their efficiency, which contributes to a buildup of toxins in your body, which leads to further deterioration of cells. It is a vicious cycle that can quickly lead to disease unless something is done to slow it down.

Keep in mind that the preceding liver example focuses on just one organ system and one set of cells in that organ. Now imagine this process occurring throughout all the organ systems of your body simultaneously. When your body is healthy, everything works together, like an orchestra. When you begin to age, everything starts to break down the same way—simultaneously. Disease follows the steady march of time along with the decline of cellular function.

Four types of cellular changes have been found to be especially significant during aging: lipid peroxidation, loss of mytochondrial function and quality, cellular receptor loss, and the loss of telomere function. Let's look at how each of these plays a role in the aging process.

Lipid Peroxidation (LPO)

Lipid peroxidation is damage caused by free radicals to cellular membranes and other molecules in the cells that contain lipids (fats). (See the inset on page 47 of Chapter 2 to learn about free radicals.) This affects membrane permeability, nutrient transport, cellular signaling, and a variety of other cell functions, eventually leading to cell death. Lipid peroxidation has been implicated in the development of atherosclerosis, asthma, Parkinson's disease, kidney damage, and many other disease states.

Loss of Mitochondrial Function and Quality

Mitochondria are organelles (specialized cellular parts) within the cells that that generate most of the chemical energy needed to fuel the cell's biochemical reactions. Basically, they take the energy we get from food and turn it into energy the cell can use. Research has shown that mitochondria also have other important functions, such as the maintenance of calcium balance in the body.

As part of the normal aging process, mitochondria decline in both quality and activity. Like lipid peroxidation, this decline, which can be hastened by poor nutrition and disease, has been associated with a number of age-related disorders.

Cellular Receptor Loss

Cellular receptors are protein molecules—found within the cells and embedded in the surface of the cells—that allow the cells to receive signals from other cells. This communication is necessary for the cells to function properly.

Unfortunately, with age, cellular receptors are either lost or become uncoupled from their specific signaling pathways. Like other cell damage, receptor signal loss leads to age-related illness.

Loss of Proper Telomere Function

The structures called *telomeres* sit at the end of the chromosomes in cells, much as protective plastic tips sit at the end of shoelaces. The job of telomeres is to stop the ends of chromosomes from fraying or sticking to each other. They also play an important role in ensuring that DNA gets copied properly when cells divide.

These structures are now known to be associated with aging. Telomeres shorten over time, and when they get too short to do their job, our cells age and stop functioning properly. Eventually, the cells stop dividing and essentially die. It has been said that telomeres act as the aging clock in every cell.

HOW TO KEEP YOUR GOLDEN YEARS GOLDEN

Just because free radicals and cellular deterioration occur naturally does not mean that you have to take them lying down. Following a healthful diet, exercising, and taking certain supplements can help your body eliminate free radicals and slow cell death. This, in turn, can delay and decrease the destructive effects of aging, reduce the incidence of illness, and enable you to grow old gracefully, whatever your racial background.

Improve Your Diet

Earlier in the chapter, you learned that free radicals are partly responsible for the deterioration of cells that is associated with aging-related problems. Harmful changes in the body's microbiome are also associated with disorders common to the aging process. Fortunately, a good diet can help address both of these problems.

As explained in Chapter 1, you can support a healthy microbiome by eating an abundant amount of vegetables, fruits, beans and legumes, and nuts—foods high in the fiber that nourishes beneficial bacteria. If possible, also add probiotic foods like yogurt and sauerkraut, which contain live bacteria. (For more about foods that support a good microbiome, see page 22.) Fruits and vegetables also contain substances known as antioxidants—vitamins A, C, and E, for instance—which neutralize those damaging free radicals. These healthful foods not only help keep you feeling younger but also help you fight obesity, diabetes, heart disease, and other health problems. A diet high in fruits, vegetables, and nuts has also been found to support the health and function of the cells' telomeres. (For more information on healthy diets, see Chapter 9.)

Get Sufficient Exercise

A good exercise program will help you delay aging by keeping your cells younger. It is known that exercise increases nitrous oxide in cells, which supports the function of mitochondria. Exercise can also maintain the health of telomeres, increasing their length and allowing them to do their job.

Exercise also improves the condition of your heart and lungs; increases blood flow to deliver nutrients to your cells and rid them of wastes; increases muscular strength, tone, endurance and fitness;

helps you maintain a normal weight; improves your coordination so that you are less likely to fall; and increases your energy levels. Your brain functions better and you have greater self-confidence and self-esteem. You won't believe how much exercise can delay many of the chronic diseases associated with old age. Here are some statistics:

- Cardiovascular disease decreases by 35 percent.
- Type 2 diabetes decreases by 40 percent.
- Colon cancer decreases by 30 percent.
- Breast cancer decreases by 20 percent.
- Depression decreases by 30 percent.
- Hip fractures decrease by 68 percent.
- Dementia decreases by 30 percent.

As you can see, adopting an exercise routine is critical if you want to have good health and age slowly. Experts recommend that you engage in moderate aerobic activity for 20 to 30 minutes a day; or, if you're engaging in vigorous aerobic activity, you exercise for a little more than 10 minutes a day. (See the inset on page 42 for an explanation of different exercise intensities.) You can also combine moderate and vigorous activity. Remember to gradually build up your time and intensity. When you're comfortable doing vigorous exercise, you may want to add strength training. You will be amazed by how much better you feel as you exercise harder and longer. This may take weeks or even months, but don't get frustrated! Even when you first begin incorporating exercise into your life, the activity will lift your spirits by releasing endorphins, the feel-good hormones.

If you are overweight or obese; if you have any kind of chronic health condition; or if you simply haven't exercised in years, be sure to check with your healthcare provider before you start an exercise program.

Take Helpful Supplements

Although your system regularly produces the protective molecules called antioxidants, which fight off the free radicals that play a major role in damaging your cells, your body does not generally produce sufficient antioxidants to defend against every free radical. Improving your diet, as described earlier in this chapter, can help provide antioxidants and can also support a healthful microbiome. But because life can get in the way of a proper meal, consider using supplements to supply antioxidants as well as probiotics. For guidance in choosing the best-quality supplements and using them effectively, see page 258. For a more complete guide to anti-aging supplements, see page 261.

Daily Multivitamins

A daily multivitamin/mineral supplement can help fill the gaps in your diet by providing many of the nutrients your body needs to function, including antioxidants such as vitamins A, C, and E. Speak to your physician about choosing the best multivitamin for you. For instance, in some cases, you may want to avoid certain nutrients, such as iron. Your physician should be able to steer you towards the right product.

Probiotics

You have learned that a healthy microbiome can help you avoid many of the problems associated with aging, including a weakened immune system. To support your microbiome, consider taking probiotic supplements, which provide good bacteria in the form of tablets, powders, or capsules. For the greatest benefit, choose a product that provides at least five different types of bacteria and more than 70 billion colonies.

Superoxide Dismutase (SOD)

The enzyme called *superoxide dismutase*, or SOD, is one of the body's most powerful antioxidants, reducing free radical damage associated with the vicious cycle of aging and a host of age-related disorders, such as heart disease, diabetes, and rheumatoid arthritis. SOD is naturally produced by your body, but when cells have been damaged over the years and can no longer generate the antioxidant enzyme in sufficient amounts, it may be time to turn to medical science, which has made it possible to take SOD through supplements. I recommend a dosage of 150 mg per day, but your doctor may suggest a slightly different amount for your individual needs.

Make Play and Recreation Part of Your Life

As George Bernard Shaw said years ago, "We don't stop playing because we grow old; we grow old because we stop playing." Shaw was onto something, because the benefits of play are many. First, playing games, creating art, and expressing creativity keep your brain active and engaged, with less memory loss. Second, when you play, you release endorphins—brain chemicals that reduce pain and lift your mood. And just as important, play reduce stress, enabling your immune system to work better. Have you had a good laugh lately? Laughter relaxes your muscles and lowers your blood pressure. And if you share a laugh with someone, you will feel closer to each other.

What, exactly, is considered "play." Stuart Brown, a retired scientist who has spent years studying the power of play, has written that what constitutes "play" varies among individuals, but that it should be about the joy of the experience rather than accomplishing a goal. As long as the activity you choose is "purposeless, fun and pleasurable," you will reap the benefits of play.

Perhaps you already have a hobby or leisure activity that makes play a part of your life. If not, here are a few suggestions: Read an interesting or funny book. Listen to music that lifts your spirits. Or play music that makes you want to dance—and then put on your dancing shoes and show your stuff! Go to a park and take a walk. Enjoy the sunshine, trees and flowers, and squirrels and rabbits scrambling around. Smile when you see a mother with her small children.

Another great option is to engage in group activities. Maybe you have friends who like to play cards or board games. Join the

YMCA and engage in some of their activities—swimming, dancing, and exercise. Or visit your library and join a book club in which everyone reads the same book and then gets together to talk about it. If you already play a musical instrument, find a group of like-minded people and make music! Remember that the music doesn't have to be perfect and professional—it's the experience that's important. The list of possibilities is endless. Choose something that makes you smile, laugh, and feel good. Remember, laughter is the best medicine.

CONCLUSION

By understanding the normal process of aging, you can see that the march of time does not have to lead to disorders that impair the quality of your life and shorten your life span. Let's keep in mind that the life span for Blacks in our country is not the same as that for Whites. While White men live 76 years and White women, 81 years; the average life span for Black men is 72 years and the average for Black women is 78 years. But it doesn't have to be that way. By making healthful changes, much of which involve diet, exercise, and other lifestyle modifications, you can improve both how you feel and how long you live. The only true killer we face is ignorance.

9

Nutrition and Diets

"The food you eat can be either the safest and most powerful
form of medicine—or the slowest form of poison."
—ANN WIGMORE

If you are to thrive and prosper, be filled with energy and purpose, and be free of the diseases that plague your community and may already affect you, *you must change your diet*. You may have grown up eating Southern and soul foods, which I understand reflect our cultural heritage and are enjoyed at our family get-togethers. I know that many of these dishes taste really good, but the fact is that they are terrible for our health. They are loaded with unhealthy fats, too much salt, too many highly processed foods, and too much sugar, all of which—separately and, even more so, in combination—make us sick and shorten our lives. As you know from previous chapters, it is our bad choice of foods that contributes to overweight and obesity, hypertension, heart disease, strokes, diabetes, and kidney disease. Plain and simple, this is the common thread that runs through all the disorders that kill our people.

In this chapter, I will give you a short history of Black nutrition and how we got where we are food-wise and health-wise. I will discuss how the state of current Southern cuisine and soul foods evolved and explain that although these methods of cooking and food preparation may be traditional, their cost to our well-being is too high.

I'll also look at the fast-food industry that targets Black families, who frequent these places because the food is tasty, filling, and cheap. Nutritious and healthy? Unfortunately, no. While you are buying and eating these harmful foods, corporate executives are raking in the money and coming up with more addictive treats designed to "hook" you and your family for life.

Finally, I'll guide you in choosing healthy, delicious foods and easy-to-follow eating plans that can help you lower your blood pressure, lose weight, and control your blood sugar. I'll even talk about ways in which you can alter some of your family favorites by adjusting the ingredients so they are more nutritious.

THE HISTORY OF BLACK NUTRITION

There was a long journey from the foods of Africa to today's African-American diets. In Africa, the natives grew several crops that provided basic starches—foods such as wheat, barley, yams, black-eyed peas, kidney beans, and lima beans—that were dietary staples. Basically, these original diets were largely vegetarian and healthy as long as there were no famines to contend with. Once Africans were captured by slave traders and placed aboard ships, they were fed twice a day on a diet of nuts or boiled Indian corn with one pint of water. It was poor in nutrition, but stable enough to last the length of their journeys across the ocean. If they refused to eat, they were flogged.

After they were removed from the ships' cargo hold and sold on the auction blocks of the Carolinas, with chains around their necks, hands, and feet, the Africans ate foods that dramatically influenced what Blacks eat today. Unlike the healthier vegetarian diet they had consumed in Africa, the food here was high in calories, fat, and salt. The kinds of meat they ate, such as bacon, are now known to cause cancer and other modern diseases. The inadequate amount of water they were given was described as a "nasty, muddy, pond of ill taste." One of the reasons that plantation owners fed pork and corn to their slaves was that they were cheap food sources and stored well for long periods of time.

But the corn was an "incomplete" protein, meaning that it did not contain all the essential building blocks (amino acids) necessary for a healthy body, and the pork was mostly fat, with very little protein. Slaves were plagued by an insufficient amount of food and water to help their bodies deal with the long, hard days of working in the fields. In nutritional terms, the staples of slaves were deficient in many vitamins and minerals—except for vitamin D, which was created by their bodies from their lengthy exposure to sunlight. However, because of the nutrient-poor foods, even the long days of sunlight did not provide quite enough of this vitamin.

Slaves learned to supplement their inadequate diet by adding the parts of animals discarded when their masters' meals were prepared, including them in their "single pot" meals whenever possible. This is where many of the foods we eat today became staples, such as pig intestines (better known as chitterlings, or chitlins), and pigs' feet and ears. Much of this was mixed with nutritious foods like collard greens, yams, black-eyed peas, and other produce. This is the origin of what we call soul food today.

Finally, when looking at the origin of Southern cooking, we must not overlook the fact that there was a considerable influence of other cultures on this style of preparing meals. The influence of the French, which led to "Creole" style; the introduction of maize (corn) by Native Americans; the spicy foods of the Caribbean; and the foods the Africans had eaten in their home lands of West and Central Africa—all were blended together to create "Southern" dishes. And for many of us, these styles of cooking were used to prepare our everyday meals as we were growing up. The recipes had been handed down for generations, and they were an essential part of our African-American culture. What we didn't know was that many of the ingredients that went into our beloved meals were, and still are, bad for us. As you read this chapter, you will learn about these harmful ingredients. Just as important, you will learn that by making a few substitutions, you can have your Mississippi Mud Cake and eat it too. (On page 175, you'll find a section on improving soul food and Southern cooking.)

THE FAST-FOOD INDUSTRY

Let's face it, fast food dominates low-income communities. Fast foods are cheap and convenient, but they are also high in all the things we need to avoid—excessive salt and sugar, white flour, and saturated fats. And, of course, they are low in fiber, fresh fruits and vegetables, and healthy foods in general.

It has been reported that fast-food companies deliberately target Black children in poor and underserved communities. In other words, it's a corporate marketing decision. Why would corporations do this? They know that the foods they serve are *addictive*—yes, fat, salt, and sugars are addictive. Once you are hooked, manufacturers can expect you to return again and again. They also know that the people in these communities won't say anything about the bad quality of the food because, up until now, most of them didn't recognize that this food was making them sick. But now you have the knowledge: You know about the harmful effects of fast food and you know that fast-food corporations are trying to addict you and your kids to inferior ingredients. With this knowledge comes the power to turn away from fast food and choose better fare that will give you and your community greater health—and better lives.

Food and Our Poor Health

In modern African-American culture, food is central to all our activities—weddings, home and social gatherings, church, and sports events. In previous chapters, we compared the incidence of various diseases in Blacks with that in Whites. What we found were much higher rates of hypertension, obesity, type 2 diabetes, kidney disease, heart disease, and strokes—and earlier deaths—in Black people. To get a better perspective on these dramatic differences in health, let's now look at the foods that United States Blacks eat compared with the foods that Whites eat.

A national study reported that on average, Blacks consume lower amounts of whole grains, fruits, and vegetable than Whites. Blacks drink higher amounts of sugar-sweetened beverages than Whites and get a larger portion of their calories from added sugars. Blacks consume more dietary cholesterol, but less fiber. Fewer Blacks than Whites meet *the Dietary Guidelines for Americans* for whole grains, fruits, vegetables, nuts, legumes, and seeds. These are the very foods that our ancestors ate in Africa before slavery! Blacks today also consume fewer daily servings of milk, cheese, and yogurt compared with Whites. The scientists also reported lower levels of potassium, magnesium, phosphorous, iron, and vitamin D in African Americans. And data shows that Blacks consume a greater percentage of calories from fast food.

So, what is it that we are missing in our food choices? The following discussions will introduce you to nutrient-rich foods that can help you stay well and feel great.

CHOOSING HEALTHY FOODS

To choose healthy foods, you must select foods with one or more of these nutritious components—protein; complex carbohydrates, which are full of fiber; essential fatty acids; and vitamins, minerals, and phytochemicals (chemicals produced by plants). These components, sometimes singly and sometimes in combination, are found in food groups such as vegetables; fruits; beans, nuts, and seeds; whole grains; lean meat, poultry, fish, and eggs; low-fat dairy and dairy alternatives; and some vegetable oils. Let's look at each of these in turn.

Vegetables

Most vegetables are naturally low in fat, calories, and sodium, and contain no cholesterol. Vegetables also provide a variety of essential nutrients, including complex carbohydrates, which are high in dietary fiber; potassium; folate; vitamins A, C, and K; and phytochemicals. There is also strong evidence that a diet rich in fruits and vegetables can lower the risk of heart disease and stroke.

Aim for about $2^1/_2$ cups of vegetables each day. (Note that 1 cup of low-salt vegetable soup counts as one serving of veggies.) Another option is to have a glass of low-salt vegetable juice.

Choose from this list of vegetables:

- Artichokes
- Asparagus
- Beets

- Bell peppers
- Bok choy
- Broccoli

- Brussels sprouts
- Cabbage
- Carrots

WHAT ARE COMPLEX CARBOHYDRATES?

Complex carbohydrates are composed of sugar molecules that are strung together in long, complex chains. Both simple and complex carbs are turned into glucose (blood sugar) in the body, where they are used as energy. But while simple carbs, like those in table sugar, are digested quickly and provide an unhealthy blast of glucose in the blood, complex carbs digest more slowly, which provides a more steady release of glucose. This helps control blood sugar levels, making foods with complex carbs ideal for people with type 2 diabetes. Foods with complex carbs typically also have more vitamins and minerals than foods containing more simple carbohydrates.

Which foods contain complex carbs? You'll find them in beans, vegetables, and whole grains, including the following:

- Barley
- Beans and legumes, such as black beans, chickpeas, and lentils
- Brown rice

- Corn
- Potatoes
- Quinoa
- Whole wheat flour, bread, and pasta

Everybody needs carbohydrates for the energy they provide for the body. But for the best nutrition and the best control of blood sugar, you'll want to stick to foods rich in complex carbohydrates.

- Cauliflower
- Celery
- Corn
- Cucumber
- Eggplant
- Garlic
- Green beans
- Jicama

- Kale
- Leeks
- Lettuce
- Onions
- Parsnips
- Peas
- Potatoes
- Rhubarb

- Scallions
- Shallots
- Spinach
- Squash
- Sweet potatoes
- Tomatoes
- Turnips
- Yams

Keep in mind that when it comes to leafy greens, the darker the green, the richer the nutrients. Skip the iceberg lettuce, and opt for richer-colored produce. Each day, aim for one to two servings of green leafy vegetables such as kale, spinach, and leafy salad greens, which supply antioxidants, vitamin C, and folic acid. Leafy greens can be steamed, used to make salads, or added to whole grain bowls. When making salads or coleslaw, mix purple cabbage with green cabbage, or use only red cabbage. Purple cabbage is ten times richer in vitamin A than green cabbage, and its high potassium content helps lower blood pressure. Purple cabbage also brightens up a plate.

Leafy greens can also be used to make smoothies. Just throw some kale or spinach in a blender along with some fruit and milk or yogurt. If you wish, add a spoonful of almond butter for protein. You won't even realize you're drinking your vegetables for breakfast.

Enjoy white potatoes or sweet potatoes only occasionally. Both types of potatoes are packed with fiber and potassium, and sweet potatoes are rich in beta-carotene, which your body converts into vitamin A. Just keep in mind that potatoes become unhealthy if you fry them or add gobs of butter, sour cream, bacon bits, and salt; or, in the case of sweet potatoes, if you add sugar and marshmallows. Bake the potatoes, add a dab of butter, and season with some herbs.

The onion family of vegetables—onions, garlic, leeks, shallots, scallions, and chives—contains sulfur compounds that act as natural blood thinners, which can help prevent blood clots. When eaten raw, these vegetables have shown the ability to lower blood pressure, too.

Eating a variety of vegetables every day will boost your nutrition while providing you with many tasty options.

WHAT ARE FLAVONOIDS?

Flavonoids are chemical compounds found naturally in fruits and vegetables, nuts, and herbs and spices, as well as in wine, tea, and dark chocolate. These compounds give fruits and vegetables their vibrant color and also increase the effectiveness of your cell's functions. Powerful antioxidants, flavonoids help your body fight off harmful free radicals and may also reduce inflammatory reactions triggered by allergens, germs, toxins, and other irritants. These helpful compounds are known to lower blood pressure and to decrease the likelihood of stroke, type 2 diabetes, and other chronic health conditions.

How can you make sure that your diet is providing you with the flavonoids you need? Clearly, loading up on fruits and vegetables is your best bet. Choose produce of different colors to make sure that you get a wide range of nutrients. And don't hesitate to season your food with herbs and spices, which are flavonoid rich. Wine, dark chocolate, and nuts should be consumed only in moderation.

Fruits

Fruits are an important part of a healthy diet. Like vegetables, they are naturally low in fat and calories, are low in sodium, and contain no cholesterol. They also supply many essential nutrients that are under-consumed in the United States, including potassium, complex carbohydrates and fiber, vitamins A and C, and folic acid.

These nutrients help maintain healthy blood pressure and normal heartbeat, reduce cholesterol, promote feelings of fullness, and encourage healthy digestion, so whenever you eat fruit, you are doing something good for your body. For instance, bananas, which are low in sodium and very high in potassium, have been found by researchers to lower blood pressure.

You should aim for about 2 cups of fruit each day. Different fruits contain different phytochemicals (there are some 5,000 different ones), including the flavonoids discussed on page 158. By choosing different kinds of fruit, you will make sure to get a greater range of phytochemicals. This will help boost your immune system, protect your cells from the damage that can lead to cancer, reduce inflammation, regulate your hormones, and otherwise maintain good body function.

Choose a rainbow of different colored fruits (and vegetables) such as red, orange, yellow, green, blue, and purple. Every day, try to include a citrus fruit such as an orange or grapefruit, which are both great sources of vitamin C and potassium. Citrus juices are also good, but keep in mind that they are high in calories and do not provide the fiber found in whole fruit.

Some of the most healthful fruits include the following:

- Apples
- Apricots
- Avocados
- Bananas
- Cantaloupe
- Casaba melons
- Cherries
- Grapefruit
- Guava
- Honeydew melons
- Kiwi
- Lemons
- Limes
- Mangos
- Nectarines
- Oranges
- Peaches
- Pears
- Pineapple
- Watermelons

For the best quality, the most nutrients, and the lowest prices, choose fruits that are "in season." The fruits should feel firm or crisp to the touch and the color should be bright. Avoid any damaged or bruised produce.

GRAPEFRUIT, FURANOCOUMARIN, AND YOUR MEDICATIONS

Grapefruit is a delicious and healthful fruit that provides vitamin C, potassium, and phytochemicals. But did you know that grapefruit should not be mixed with certain drugs that are prescribed for heart disease, high blood pressure, and some other disorders? In fact, the instructions that accompany many medications specificially tell you *not* to eat grapefruit or drink grapefruit juice while taking the medication. This is because grapefruit contains natural compounds called furanocoumarins that can interfere with the body's conversion of the medication to its active forms and prevent it from being broken down for elimination from the body. If this occurs, the metabolites of the medication, which can be toxic, accumulate in the blood, potentially causing problems. The list below contains some of the medications affected by grapefruit. If you are not sure if the medications you are taking would interact with grapefruit, speak to your pharmacist for more information.

- Some statin drugs taken to lower cholesterol, such as Zocor (simvastatin) and Lipitor (atorvastatin).

- Some drugs that treat high blood pressure, such as Procardia and Adalat CC (both nifedipine).

- Some immunosupressive drugs, such as Sandimmune and Neoral (both cyclosporine).

- Some anti-anxiety drugs, such as buspirone.

- Some corticosteroids that treat Crohn's disease or ulcerative colitis, such as Entocort EC and Uceris (both budesonide).

- Some drugs that treat abnormal heart rhythms, such as Pacerone and Nexterone (both amiodarone).

- Some antihistamines, such as Allegra (fexofenadine).

Beans, Nuts, and Seeds

Beans are among the most ancient of foods and are also the most commonly eaten foods in the world. If you are confused about the differences between beans and legumes, keep in mind that legumes are a class of vegetables that include beans, peas, and related vegetables. All of these foods are truly super foods. They are low in price but high in vitamins, minerals, protein, essential fatty acids, fiber, and a variety of phytochemicals. Legumes could actually be listed as both vegetables and proteins—that's how beneficial they are. They are also known to decrease insulin levels, improve metabolic syndrome and pre-diabetes, lower body weight, lower cholesterol, and reduce blood pressure. That's pretty amazing!

I recommend that you eat a serving of cooked beans—about 1/2 cup each—and/or a bean dish several times a week. Beans can be used in salads, soups, side dishes, and entrées. When choosing dried beans, make sure they are firm and without mold. Buy in bulk if you wish, because beans store well. Beans that you cook yourself are the healthiest because you can control the amount of salt being used, but if you prefer the convenience of canned beans, choose low-sodium brands or place the beans in a sieve and rinse them thoroughly under cold running water to wash away as much sodium as possible.

Here are some common beans that you may wish to add to your diet:

- Black beans
- Black-eyed peas
- Cannellini beans
- Chickpeas
- Fava beans
- Kidney beans
- Lentils
- Lima beans
- Navy beans
- Pinto beans
- Northern beans
- Peas
- Red beans
- Soybeans

Nuts and seeds are little packets chock-full of important nutrients. They are high in protein, the B vitamins, vitamin E, beta-carotene, calcium, copper, magnesium, phosphorous, selenium, essential fatty acids, and fiber. Nuts have been found to lower cholesterol and triglycerides, decrease fasting blood sugar, decrease inflammation, and reduce the risk of heart disease.

Nuts should be purchased in their raw, unsalted form and stored in a cool, dry place. Roasted nuts should be avoided, as high heat destroys some of their nutrients. Roasted nuts can also have a lot of salt added to them. Eat about a handful a day, but remember that 80 percent of a nut is made up of fat, and even though most of this fat is beneficial, it still means nuts are high in calories, with about 260 calories in $1^1/_2$ ounces. So eat nuts only in moderation.

Here are some common nuts and seeds that you might enjoy:

- Almonds
- Brazil nuts
- Cashews
- Chia seeds
- Flaxseeds
- Hazelnuts
- Hemp seeds
- Pecans
- Pine nuts
- Pistachios
- Pumpkin seeds
- Sesame seeds
- Sunflower seeds
- Walnuts

Whole Grains

Whole grains are naturally high in fiber, helping you feel full and satisfied. They are also an important source of many nutrients, including a number of B vitamins (thiamin, riboflavin, niacin, and folate), vitamin E, iron, copper, magnesium, selenium, zinc, essential fatty acids, and phytochemicals. Because of these nutrients, whole grains have been linked to a lower risk of heart disease, diabetes, certain cancers, and other health problems. Why should you eat whole grains instead of refined grains, like white rice? When grains are refined, they are stripped of the nutrient-rich bran, which supplies B vitamins, iron, copper, zinc, phytochemicals, and more.

Try to eat five to six half-cup servings of whole grains, such as brown rice, each day. Also look for whole-grain pastas, crackers, and dense whole-grain breads. When buying whole grains, make sure the package says "100% Whole Grain." When buying whole-grain breads, make sure that the first ingredient is whole wheat or another whole grain. Common grains include:

- Amaranth
- Faro
- Wheat berries
- Barley
- Oats and oatmeal
- Wild rice
- Brown rice
- Quinoa
- Whole wheat
- Bulgur wheat
- Rye

Lean Meat, Poultry, Fish, and Eggs

For a balanced diet, men need about 56 grams of protein each day, while women need about 46 grams per day. When you eat foods containing protein, your body breaks them down into smaller units called *amino acids*, which are referred to as the "building blocks" of protein. Your body uses these amino acids to make the special proteins used to repair cells, to make new cells, and to grow and develop normally.

Of the twenty amino acids needed by the body, your body can make eleven but must get nine of them from dietary sources. All nine are found in meat, poultry, eggs, and fish. Although these are all sources of *complete protein*, complete proteins can also be found in non-animal sources, including quinoa and soybeans. Nuts, leafy green vegetables, and most grains and legumes do not contain all nine essential amino acids, but if you combine these foods within a day's meals, you will get complete proteins—without any saturated fat or cholesterol. In other words, you don't need to get all your protein from animal sources.

Meat and Chicken

Although red meat is an important source of protein, essential amino acids, vitamins, and minerals, it also contains more cholesterol and saturated fats than chicken, fish, or vegetables. A high consumption of red meat has been associated with a greater risk of stroke, cardiovascular death, and certain types of cancer. Eat lean beef and other red meats sparingly. Instead, eat poultry—chicken and turkey—choosing white meat over dark and removing the skin. Sauté, grill, or roast the poultry rather than frying it. Aim for one 4-ounce portion of meat or chicken a day.

The consumption of processed meat such as ham, sausage, bacon, luncheon meat, and hot dogs increases the risk of major age-related diseases, including stroke. The reason is not clear, but it may be due to the use of sodium nitrite, a preservative. Save these processed foods for special times—say, a hot dog at the ballpark or a slice of ham on Easter. Do not make them part of your everyday meals.

Eggs

Eggs are another source of protein and many other nutrients. The yolk is also rich in phytochemicals, and some eggs contain a small amount of omega-3 fatty acids. (Check the package.) Yes, eggs are one of the richest dietary sources of cholesterol, but they also contain nutrients that may lower the risk of heart disease and stroke.

For the greatest health benefits, don't scramble or fry your eggs, because the high heat and oxygen in the air damage the cholesterol, causing it to be harmful. Instead, serve your eggs soft-boiled, poached, or hard-boiled. If you are healthy, eat up to two whole eggs a day. If you have health problems, ask your healthcare provider if you should limit your consumption of eggs.

Seafood

Seafood is a great source of protein and healthy omega-3 fatty acids. Aim for two to three servings of seafood each week. (One serving consists of 3 ounces of fish.) Avoid frying fish. Instead, it can be sautéed in a little olive oil, baked, or broiled. Good seafood options include omega-3-rich fish such as albacore tuna, salmon, sardines, herring, and other fatty fish. Cod, catfish, clams, scallops, and shrimp are also excellent choices, even if they are not great sources of omega-3s. Let's not forget that fish is a major source of vitamin D_3. Keep in mind that most of the vitamin D found in foods, other than fish, requires conversion in the body to the effective form of vitamin D_3.

Dairy Products and Alternatives

Dairy products provide many important nutrients, including protein, probiotics, and vitamins and minerals—calcium, vitamin A, vitamin B_2, vitamin B_3, vitamin B_{12}, vitamin D, calcium, phosphorous, and potassium. The USDA recommends that adults have three servings of dairy each day, with a serving being one cup of milk, one cup of yogurt, or $1^1/_2$ ounces of cheese. The nutrients in dairy are vital for the health and maintenance of your body and are particularly necessary for keeping bones strong. Dairy products are also associated with better management of blood pressure and blood sugar levels.

Although we have assumed for decades that the fat in dairy is unhealthy, a growing body of scientific evidence suggests that dairy fat does not increase the risk of cardiovascular disease. Recent studies have found that whole-fat dairy does not cause weight gain, and that it improves body composition by increasing lean body mass and reducing body fat. Yogurt consumption reduces weight gain; fermented dairy, including cheese, lowers cardiovascular risk; and both yogurt and cheese protect against type 2 diabetes. However, always keep recommended portions in mind. Too much of nearly any food can cause weight gain and the problems that accompany it.

Those who avoid milk and other dairy products, whether due to allergy, lactose intolerance, or personal preference, should try to get similar nutrition from dairy alternatives, which include almond milk, coconut milk, rice milk, soy milk, hemp milk, and oat milk. Just be aware that milk substitutes usually do not have the same nutrients as dairy milk. With the exception of soy milk, they may not offer complete protein—meaning that they lack some essential amino acids. They also may provide little or no calcium, and they may contain added sugar. Be sure to check both the ingredients lists and the Nutrition Facts label so that you know what you're getting. Some brands, for instance, fortify their products with calcium.

Some dairy products are very high in saturated fat. For this reason, sour cream, cream cheese, heavy cream, and buttermilk should be eaten rarely or only in fat-reduced forms. Butter is made from animal fat, so it contains saturated fat. If you ask most doctors, they will tell you to replace your butter with margarine, but the truth is that there is no good evidence that butter increases the risk of heart attack or stroke. If you like olive oil, definitely use it instead of butter. If you prefer butter, use small amounts rather than slathering it on potatoes and bread.

Vegetable Oils and Dressings

The fatty acids and other nutrients found in certain vegetable oils are protective against a variety of cardiovascular diseases. Generally, two to three servings of vegetable oil a day—with each serving being about one tablespoon—are considered beneficial.

Extra virgin olive oil is an especially healthful choice. While olive oil does not contain a large amount of omega-3 fatty acids, it does contain high levels of oleic acid, an omega-9 fatty acid that has been associated with the reduction of inflammation. It also is a good source of vitamin E and provides vitamins A and K, iron, calcium, magnesium, and potassium, as well as strong antioxidants. Olive oil has been found to lower blood pressure, help control blood sugar and insulin sensitivity, lower bad cholesterol, and boost good cholesterol.

Other healthy vegetable oil options include canola and walnut oils, both of which are high in omega-3 fatty acids. Avoid corn, soy, safflower, sunflower, and peanut oils because they are high in essential omega-6 fatty acids. Although most Americans don't get adequate amounts of omega-3s, they get more than enough omega-6s, which are found in many processed foods.

DIETS FOR A LONGER, HEALTHIER LIFE

There are all kinds of diets available—some to help you lose weight, others to reduce your risk of cardiovascular disease, others to lower your blood pressure, others to help you adopt a vegetarian diet. No matter which diet you decide to adopt, it's vital to eat only nutritionally superior foods and, in most cases, it's important to consume fewer calories. Unless you are a vegetarian, it's recommended that you have these basic foods and beverages every day:

- Fruits and vegetables

- Seafood, lean meats and poultry, eggs, beans, and/or unsalted nuts or seeds

- Fat-free or low-fat milk and milk products, including fortified soy beverages

- Whole grains such as oatmeal, whole-wheat bread, and brown rice

Below are several different diet plans. I will tell you briefly about each diet and then lead you to helpful websites in the Resources section, so that you can learn more about any diet that sounds good to you. Keep in mind that literally hundreds of different diets are being promoted every day. I have selected the ones I think provide the most benefits and have been shown to work. If you choose to follow another diet, just make sure it provides you with all the nutrients you need and protects your microbiome. (We discuss that on page 172.) Hopefully, over time, you will find an eating plan that you enjoy and are able to stay with for years.

We'll start with the American Heart Association Diet, but keep in mind that the other eating plans we discuss will also help prevent cardiovascular disease.

The American Heart Association (AHA) Diet

The American Heart Association Diet was created as an eating plan that reduces the risk of cardiovascular disease, such as heart disease and stroke. Over the years, it has evolved to also include good general lifestyle habits and goals. One goal, for instance, is to use both calorie counting and exercise so that you use up at least as many calories as you take in. Another goal is to live tobacco-free by avoiding both smoking and exposure to secondhand smoke.

The AHA's major dietary recommendation is to eat a variety of nutritious foods from all the food groups: fruits and vegetables, whole grains, low-fat dairy products, skinless poultry and fish, nuts and legumes, and non-tropical vegetable oils. The diet

LIMIT ADDED SUGARS

Many of us grew up drinking sugar-sweetened beverages and enjoying sweet desserts and treats. Now, health experts know that an excess of sweetened foods and beverages can lead to a variety of problems, from weight gain to poor blood sugar control to high blood pressure to an increased risk of heart disease. For these reasons, added sugar should be kept to a minimum. This means not only staying away from the sugar bowl but also avoiding soda, fruit drinks, sports drinks, and energy drinks.

At first, you may find that you don't feel good when you give up all the sweet "goodies." This is because you are actually addicted to sugar. Yes, sugar is addictive, which is why giant food companies spend millions of dollars adding sugar to foods. The sugar keeps everyone coming back for more. Although you should stay away from sugar-sweetened products, you should also steer clear of artificially sweetened foods and beverages. These foods are created to taste great, but they are really bad for you and, as strange as it might seem, they do not result in weight loss. Instead, they increase your cravings for sugar.

How much sugar is okay? In a perfect world, no one would eat plain granulated sugar or sugar additives. But because these sweeteners are baked into our food products, avoiding sugar in today's world is difficult. The American Heart Association sets a daily limit of 6 teaspoons (24 grams) of sugar for women and 9 teaspoons (36 grams) of sugar for men. It's easy to keep track of what you are adding in the kitchen or at the table, but for products you buy at the store, look at the Nutrition Facts label for "Added Sugars" and "Total Sugars." Keep in mind that 4 grams equal 1 teaspoon.

It is also a good habit to read the Ingredients listing on any product you buy. The manufacturer must list the individual ingredients in order of amount, from the largest amount to the smallest. Be aware, though, that most companies use more than one type of sugary ingredient, so even if sugar is not one of the first ingredients named, there may in fact be lots of sugar in the product. The most common culprits are high-fructose corn syrup and various fruit concentrates, but there are many more. And if you think it's wrong to include all these different sugars, you are right.

recommends that you limit saturated fat; eliminate trans fat; reduce sodium to no more than 2,300 milligrams of sodium per day; and greatly reduce red meat, sweets, and sugar-sweetened beverages. Also eat a variety of fish, especially oily fish containing omega-3 fatty acids, twice each week; and eat limited amounts of lean meats. Be sure to maintain a healthy weight, and limit alcohol to one daily drink for a woman and two drinks for a man.

While the goal of the AHA Diet is to reduce cardiovascular disease, it also reduces risk factors such as obesity, unhealthy cholesterol, and high triglycerides; lowers blood pressure; and helps to normalize blood glucose levels. For more information, visit the website provided in the Resources section (see page 285).

The Mediterranean Diet

The Mediterranean Diet originated in the 1960s in Spain, Italy, Greece, and other countries bordering the Mediterranean Sea. At that time, doctors and scientists began to observe that these populations were healthier and had much less heart disease than other groups. Today, the Mediterranean Diet is characterized by a high consumption of vegetables and olive oil and a moderate consumption of protein. The foundation is vegetables, fruits, herbs, nuts, beans, and whole grains. (Doesn't this sound like what our ancestors ate in Africa?) The diet contains a moderate amount of sodium because of traditional foods such as olives and cheese. This diet is celebrated worldwide and has been shown to reduce the incidence of heart disease and stroke, type 2 diabetes, certain cancers, and depression, and improve mental and physical health. For more information, see page 286 of the Resources section.

The DASH Diet (Dietary Approaches to Stop Hypertension)

Based on studies sponsored by the National Heart, Lung, and Blood Institute (NHLBI), the DASH Diet was designed to help treat or prevent high blood pressure. It includes lots of whole grains, fruits, vegetables, and low-fat dairy products, as well as some fish, poultry, and legumes. Small amounts of nuts and seeds are included a few times a week. Foods that are high in saturated fat and cholesterol are to be eaten less frequently, and trans fats are to be avoided altogether. There is both a standard DASH Diet and a lower-sodium version.

How does the DASH Diet fight hypertension? It contains plentiful amounts of potassium, magnesium, calcium, fiber, and protein—all nutrients associated with lower blood pressure. Scientific studies have shown that DASH lowers blood pressure effectively in pre-hypertensive and hypertensive adults, both Black and White—but especially in Blacks. Other studies have concluded that the DASH Diet also lowers levels of cholesterol, improves the action of insulin, and reduces weight. For more information on the DASH Diet, see page 286 of the Resoureces section.

A Vegetarian Diet

A vegetarian diet consists mainly or exclusively of plant foods—much like the diet our ancestors ate in Africa. Because they are lower in or free of animal products, these diets are low in total and saturated fat and cholesterol. Refined carbs and highly processed items should be avoided.

Different people adopt a vegetarian diet for different reasons. Some object to the use of animals raised and killed for our plea-sure. Others have chronic diseases and have heard that this diet can help them lose weight, lower their blood pressure and cholesterol levels, and manage their diabetes. Once they try the vegetarian way of living, they sometimes find that they have new energy and enthusiasm for life.

According to the Mayo Clinic, "a vegetarian diet is a healthy way to meet your nutritional needs." There are at least four differ-ent plans:

- A *lacto vegetarian diet* excludes meat, fish, poultry, and eggs, but allows dairy products.

- An *ovo-vegetarian diet* excludes meat, poultry, seafood, and dairy products, but allows eggs.

- A *lacto-ovo vegetarian* diet excludes meat, fish, and poultry, but allows dairy products and eggs.

- A *vegan diet* excludes all animal products, including meat, fish, poultry, eggs, dairy, and even honey.

The vegetarian diet you choose will determine its nutritional content. A meal plan made up of nutritious plant foods can help you lose weight and reduce your risk of heart disease, diabetes, and some cancers. However, it does raise some nutritional concerns:

- If you avoid milk, you will get less vitamin D from your diet, although some alternatives to cow's milk, such as some soy or rice milks, are fortified with vitamin D. However, you will still probably need to take a vitamin D supplement.

- Vitamin B_{12} is necessary to produce red blood cells to prevent anemia. It can be difficult to get enough B_{12} on a vegan diet, so consider taking a supplement.

- Omega-3 fatty acids are critical for your heart and brain to function well. Diets that don't include fish and eggs are generally low in omega-3s. Canola oil, walnuts, ground flaxseed, and soybeans are good vegetarian sources of short-chain fatty acids, so you can add those to your diet. Also ask your healthcare provider if you need to take vegetarian omega-3 fatty acids in supplement form.

- Make sure that you consume foods containing iron and zinc. Dried beans and peas, enriched cereals, whole-grain products, dark green leafy vegetables, and dried fruit are good sources of these two nutrients. However, both iron and zinc from plants are more difficult to absorb. Consider taking a multivitamin-and-mineral supplement that provides these nutrients.

- Iodine is an important nutrient because it is a component of thyroid hormones. Vegans may not get enough iodine, so buy iodized salt and use it whenever you use salt. You need only about a quarter of a teaspoon a day.

Eating a vegetarian diet can be healthy as long as you are knowledgeable about all its components. For more information, go to page 287 of the Resources section.

PROBIOTIC FOODS

If you read Chapter 1, you know that a healthy *microbiome*—the colonies of good bacteria found largely within your gastrointestinal tract—is needed to keep your body strong and healthy. The microbes in the human body carry on a myriad of tasks, including generating nutrition by breaking down foods, synthesizing some vitamins, regulating your metabolism, detoxifying cancer-causing substances, and more. (For more information about the significance of these microbes, see page 15 in Chapter 1.) Because these bacteria are so important, *probiotic foods*—foods that contain live healthful bacteria—should be incorporated in every diet. These foods include the following:

- **CHEESE:** the best cheeses are gouda, mozzarella, cheddar, and cottage cheese.

- **FERMENTED PICKLES:** look for pickles made without vinegar, as vinegar pickles do not have probiotic effects.

- **KEFIR:** a fermented milk drink made using a culture of yeasts and bacteria.

- **KIMCHI:** a traditional side dish of salted and fermented vegetables, such as napa cabbage and Korean radish.

- **KOMBUCHA TEA:** a fermented, lightly effervescent, sweetened black or green tea drink that is rich in probiotics.

- **NATTO:** a traditional Japanese food made from fermented soybeans.

- **SAUERKRAUT:** finely shredded fermented cabbage.

- **TEMPEH:** a fermented soybean product.

- **TRADITIONAL BUTTERMILK:** a drink made from fermented milk or cream.

● **YOGURT:** fermented milk.

Add probiotic foods to your diet as often as possible. If few of these foods appeal to you, consider adding probiotic supplements to your daily routine. For best results, choose a product that provides at least five different types of bacteria and more than 70 billion colonies. Anything less is a waste of your money.

FASTING

Regardless of the diet you adopt, fasting is often recommended as a good way to lose weight, detoxify (remove the toxins from) your cells, lower blood glucose and cholesterol levels, and reduce blood pressure. I recommend intermittent fasting. According to the *New England Journal of Medicine*, "Preclinical studies and clinical trials have shown that intermittent fasting has benefits for many health conditions, such as obesity, diabetes mellitus, cardiovascular disease, cancers, and neurologic disorders. Animal models show that intermittent fasting improves health throughout the life span."

Intermittent fasting has three variations from which you can choose:

1. **THE ALTERNATE DAYS METHOD.** Using this method, you fast every other day.

2. **THE 5:2 METHOD.** In this method, you fast for two days and eat for five days. You then repeat.

3. **THE DAILY TIME-RESTRICTED METHOD.** Using this method, you determine a window of time each day to eat and then fast for twelve to sixteen hours of the same day, every day. In the regimen I use, we eat between 12:00 noon and 9:00 pm. This gives us a nine-hour window in which we eat followed by fifteen hours of fasting. Note that much of the time we're fasting, we're also sleeping, which makes it easier.

One of the basic goals of fasting, in addition to detoxifying the body, is to switch the body from burning sugar as fuel to using ketones. Ketones are a metabolite made of fatty acids. Burning ketones instead of glucose is beneficial to the brain.

Do not eliminate fluids during your fast because your body will not tolerate it. The body requires water and is actually made up of 70-percent water. Therefore, you must always remain hydrated whether or not you are fasting. Ideally, to maintain normal metabolism, your daily fluid intake should be thirty-two to sixty-four ounces of water. To add some flavor to your water, consider a twist of lemon or lime.

I do not include juices in my fasts because they are full of sugar. Sports and energy drinks are often sweetened, too. Let's also understand that drinking water is only part of your daily fluid intake. The rest comes from food. A good healthy diet contains foods that are full of water—foods like fruits and vegetables—and provides about 70 percent of all the fluids you take in.

Hmmm. Notice I never said that you should include Coke or Pepsi—or any soda, regardless of brand—in your diet. Nor did I suggest beer or another alcohol. Okay, every now and then, a soda or beer won't hurt. On special occasions, or if you're hanging out with your friends, enjoy. Then get back to your routine. Take pleasure in the good things in life, but do what you can to maintain your health.

A Word of Caution

While you are detoxifying your body through fasting, do not be surprised if you begin feeling ill. Remember that toxins are stored in your body, usually in fat cells. When you fast, you begin moving the toxins from the storage reservoir into the bloodstream. These toxins will be in different forms, and some will make their way to the brain. This can make you feel dizzy or perhaps nauseous.

In the Resources section, you will find several sites that provide specific details on carrying out intermittent fasting. Find the one that you think might work best for you. Just be aware there are several other variations of this fast as well.

MAKING SOUL FOOD AND
SOUTHERN COOKING HEALTHIER

You may be thinking, "I confess. I live to eat. The food I grew up with—that my mother and both my grandmothers served—is what I want!" Or you may think, "I know I need to lose weight, but I just have to have some familiar foods, too. Are there ways to improve those foods nutritionally without cutting them out?" Yes, I will give you some suggestions, and you can find online articles and books to improve the nutrition of these foods you love. (See page 289 of the Resources section.)

To be clear, everything eaten and included in the Southern cooking style isn't bad. Collard greens and its cousins have been eaten for centuries and have great nutritional value. They provide considerable vitamins, minerals, and fiber, but just not enough to overcome all the ingredients that people generally add when preparing them and the preparation methods themselves. As you know, Southern meals and soul foods are often high in added fats, fried food, processed meats, and sugary beverages—that wonderful iced tea and lemonade that's laced with a ton of sugar. But that doesn't mean that you have to give these foods up, because they can all be made to contain less fat, sugar, and salt and to be higher in nutrients. Here are some tips:

- One simple way to improve your diet is to reduce all the salt you use in the kitchen and add at the table. Begin by substituting herbs and spices for the salt used during the cooking process. Like sugar, salt is addictive, so at first, you may miss all the saltiness. But before long, you will have reset your taste buds and will find heavily salted foods inedible.

- Also decrease the amount of sugar you use. Make that peach cobbler, but use much less sugar than usual and depend more on the sweetness of the peaches.

- Use white whole wheat flour instead of white flour. White whole wheat flour is great because it has the benefits of whole grains but a texture more like that of white flour.

- Use canola oil instead of butter when preparing biscuits or other baked goods. Considering that you've decreased the sugar and replaced the flour with a whole-grain variety, you'll be serving much healthier treats.

- Make your cornbread using whole cornmeal instead of refined cornmeal.

- Don't give up beans like black-eyed peas. They are very nutrient-dense, meaning they are relatively low in calories but high in nutrients. But instead of using pork and bacon, try a vegetarian version. (There are many online.) If you insist on keeping the bacon and pork, use much less than usual and reduce or eliminate any salt.

- Collard greens are nutrient-dense, too—loaded with vitamins A, C, and K and with iron and magnesium—so don't eliminate them from your diet. Again, reduce the bacon or make a vegetarian version of the greens.

- Candied yams and sweet potatoes are packed with fiber, potassium, and manganese. It's just the "candied" part of this dish that is a problem. Try greatly reducing the sugar and see if you can get by with less or none. Or enjoy a baked sweet potato with a little butter and cinnamon.

- Instead of making your usual fried chicken or fish, prepare the batter with white whole wheat flour and bake the chicken or fish instead of frying it.

- If your iced tea and lemonade are highly sweetened, try learning to enjoy iced tea without any sugar and make your lemonade with far less sugar.

The above are some examples of adaptations that will allow you to enjoy healthier versions of traditional dishes. Experiment with your family's favorites. Share your recipes with friends. Tell your children why you are changing some of your recipes and teach them all about nutrition. Some recipes are impossible to make healthy, so save them for special occasions like birthdays, Christmas, and other special times of the year. Then don't stuff yourself with seconds—or thirds!

Yes, this is a departure from your cultural eating style. Remember that it has not been abandoned altogether. Instead, the dishes have been made more nutritious so that our families live longer, healthier lives.

WHERE DO YOU GO FROM HERE?

The next steps are yours. The first and biggest step is to decide that you and your family will start eating healthier foods. No doubt, this may strain your finances—fresh fruit costs more than fast food—but let's put this in perspective. You can invest in better food choices now, or you can pay for medical care and prescriptions later on. It's all about the choices you make.

The poor choice is to continue eating the same way you have eaten your whole life. The better choice is to make at least some dietary changes—changes that will provide you with the nutrients you need for good health and eliminate foods and preparation methods that will block your progress. Of course, not everyone who is Black eats poorly. Perhaps you are someone who recognizes how important nutrition is. Good for you. Unfortunately, based on the statistics, too many of our brothers and sisters do not.

CONCLUSION

A healthy way of eating is not going to cure you of every illness or pain you may be experiencing, and it will probably not take the place of any medication you're now taking to manage a health disorder. However, what good nutrition can do is pretty amazing. Consider this:

- It can lower your odds of suffering from a heart attack, stroke, diabetes, cancer, kidney disease, obesity, and a dozen other terrible health disorders.

- It can raise your body's immunity levels to fight off infections and diseases.

- It can extend your life so that you can see your grandchildren grow up.

- It can help you avoid becoming just another statistic—another African American who died too early.

I clearly understand that changing the way you eat is not necessarily going to be easy. Yes, it takes willpower, but in many cases, it may take a lot more. Fresh wholesome food may not be all that close to where you live. Maybe the extra cost of buying better food is out of your price range. Or maybe you're just hooked on the junk food you eat every day. You may have lots of reasons—excuses—to avoid changing your diet, but look at it this way: Our slave ancestors were forced to eat the "master's" garbage they were given. And now, generations later, too many of us seem to have not broken the habit of eating food that is bad for our health and the health of our children.

While it's easy to see the ugly face of racism, we seem to be blind to something that is just as bad—a diet that robs us of our health, diminishes the quality of our lives, and steals years that should belong to us. While racism is not going to change overnight, you have it in your power to eat better right now. It may take some work at first, but once you begin to experience the benefits of a good diet, you will see that it was well worth the effort.

10

Environmental Health

"Clean communities, healthy citizens."
—Lailah Gifty Akita

Your environment is the entire world you live in. It includes the air you breathe, the food you eat, the water you drink, and the substances you come in contact with at home, at work, and at play. Obviously, we are all subject to the impact our environment has on our bodies, our minds, and our health. And as I see it, we have two distinct environments to consider. The first is our *external environment*. That's the one everyone thinks of when they hear the word environment. It's the world we live in—all the objects, chemicals, and compounds we are exposed to daily. The second is our *internal environment*. That refers to all the structures, organs, and chemicals inside our body—and, as we will see, it is directly impacted by our external environment. These are the inescapable elements of our entire existence, as they will be for our children and our children's children.

It is important to understand that our exposure to the elements of our environment does not begin at birth. It begins as we develop in our mother's womb. As a fetus, for nine months we are "surrounded" by our mother's internal environment, an environment over which she has little control.

For many years, we have heard a lot about the dangers of climate change and the pollution in our water and air, and how it can destroy our planet. The truth is that our ancestors have been exposed to thousands of toxic chemical for centuries. From the lead-lined viaducts that transported water throughout the Roman Empire to the lead pipes that brought water into the homes of people living in Flint, Michigan—from the Love Canal area in New York that was built on a toxic chemical dump site to the asbestos dust coming out of the mines in Libby, Montana. Historically, we have all been subject to environmental poisons.

However, when you look closely at the statistics, for decades—if not centuries—it has been the Black communities that have suffered the most from the harmful environments in the United States. The environment has been one of the biggest factors that has caused illnesses and complicated pre-existing diseases in our communities. It has proven to be a destroyer of life, and yet too few of us actually are aware of it. This is what this chapter is all about. It was designed to help you recognize the environmental problems around you and then do what you can do fix them.

ENVIRONMENTAL HEALTH AFFECTS US FROM THE START OF LIFE

Environmental health is the branch of health that focuses on the relationship between people and their environment. What you need to understand is that the environment has the ability to make you sick and even kill you. Even worse, by the time we take our first breath, we are likely to have been poisoned in some way. If you think that's too strong a statement to make, consider the following findings of a landmark study done by the Environmental Working Group in collaboration with Commonweal on the effect of environmental exposure on fetal growth.

In the Environmental Working Group study, researchers found an average of 200 industrial pollutants and chemicals—and as many as 287 chemicals—present in umbilical cord blood taken from ten babies in the United States in 2004. The blood contained pesticides, consumer product ingredients, and waste products from the burning of gasoline, coal, and garbage. Of the chemicals found, we know that 180 of them cause cancer in humans or animals, 217 are toxic to the brain and nervous system, and 208 cause birth defects.

As you can imagine, a toxic fetal environment can take its toll on a child's health from the beginning, and may affect him for years to come. And, of course, if unborn babies are being exposed to such a toxic environment, so are all the people around them. Which groups live in the most toxic areas of this country? If your answer is "communities of color," you are correct.

POLLUTION INEQUITY

If your home or job is located near a chemical factory, a polluted lake or river, or a coal burning plant, you are likely to be in a highly toxic environment. If so, you are also likely to be a victim of *pollution inequity*, a term used to describe the fact that Blacks, Hispanics, and some other minorities are disproportionately exposed to different forms of pollution, including air pollution, pollutants in our food, and pollutants in the places we call home. Let's look at each of these forms.

The Air We Breathe

Most of us assume that inner city air is more polluted, and a recent study conducted by researchers at the University of Minnesota and the University of Washington bears this out. The researchers looked at tiny particles called PM2.5 found in polluted air. (*PM* stands for particulate matter, and *2.5* means the particles are smaller than 2.5 micrometers.) While you may have never heard of PM2.5—which can be made of hundreds of different chemicals—each year, it is a major factor in more than 100,000 deaths from heart attacks, strokes, lung cancer, and other diseases. It can also trigger asthma attacks, difficulty breathing, decreased lung function, and irregular heartbeats.

Studies have found that Blacks daily inhale about 56 percent more of this particle than other toxins. And compared with White areas, Black areas have higher PM2.5 concentrations. Add to that fact that there are thousands of other chemicals found in the air—coming from car exhaust, factories, ash, and soot—in these same Black neighborhoods.

Another report, *Fumes Across the Fence-Line*, sponsored by the NAACP, looked at the health impacts of air pollutants from oil and gas facilities. These were the report's findings:

- More than 1 million African Americans live within a half mile of existing natural gas facilities, and the number is growing every year.

- As a result, many African American communities face an elevated risk of cancer due to toxic emissions from natural gas development: Over 1 million African Americans live in counties that face a cancer risk above EPA's level of concern from toxins emitted by natural gas facilities.

- The air in many African-American communities violates air-quality standards for ozone smog. Rates of asthma are relatively high in African-American communities. And, as a result of ozone increases due to natural gas emissions during the summer season, African-American children are burdened by 138,000 asthma attacks and 101,000 lost school days each year.

- More than 6.7 million African Americans live in the 91 counties with oil refineries.

Considering that the oil and gas industry dumps 9 million tons of methane and toxic pollutants like benzene into our air each year, you can see that things are not getting better.

The Food We Eat

The limited availability of healthful food in minority areas, first discussed in Chapter 2 (see page 32), only adds to the residents' exposure to environmental toxins. Much of the foods available in underserved communities—often referred to as *food deserts*—are high in contaminants like pesticides and herbicides, as well as the antibiotics and hormones used to produce meats. And don't forget the artificial flavors, colors, and preservatives deliberately used to make processed foods taste good, look good, and have a longer shelf life. Of course, unlike the other contaminants in our foods, these additives must be listed on the products' ingredients labels.

The food stores in underserved communities also offer fewer organically grown fresh fruits and vegetables, as well as other organic products. All of these factors continually add to our communities' burden of toxins. Is it any wonder that infant mortality rates are greater for African Americans than for any other minority group in the nation—or why we generally get sicker earlier in our lives and remain so? The problem is that too many of us aren't aware of the causes of our health problems.

Pollution in Our Homes

In the same way we are not aware of the toxins in our food, we are often not aware of the pollution found in our homes and work areas. The actual materials used to build the structures where we live, the paint we put on the walls, the carpet we use on the floors—all of these materials, and many more, can actually impair our health. Because most of us spend more time at home than we do anywhere else, this is a very important aspect of our environment. The next portion of this chapter looks at the potential threats you may find in your home and how you can eliminate them.

IT BEGINS AT HOME

While we may have little or no ability to change certain environmental problems, such as the air we breathe when we walk throughout our neighborhoods, we can do a great deal to make our homes safer. The first step is to understand the biggest threats that may be present: asbestos, lead, mold, plastics, and volatile organic compounds (VOCs). These different substances can affect us in different ways, and some are easier to eliminate than others. Once we understand what these substances are, where they can be found, and why they pose a danger, we can start removing them and make our home a true sanctuary.

Asbestos

Asbestos is naturally-occurring fibrous silicate mineral that has long been used to make inexpensive fire-resistant building materials.

SICK BUILDING SYNDROME

Sick building syndrome is a term used to describe a situation in which a building's occupants experience symptoms of ill health that appear to be associated with time spent in the building and not to a specific disease. Symptoms can include headaches, sinus problems, runny and irritated eyes and nose, throat irritation and tightness, fatigue, dizziness, and nausea. The building may be a residence or a place of work.

How do you know if you are suffering from sick building syndrome? The test is simple. When you are in the building, your symptoms are evident. When you leave the building, the symptoms generally clear up within a few hours. How do you learn the specific cause of the problem? The most common contaminant of indoor air is volatile organic compounds, or VOCs, which are discussed on page 190. Other culprits can include contaminants that come in from the outside, such as motor vehicle exhaust that enters the building through windows or vents; biological contaminants such as pollen, bacteria, viruses, fungus, and molds; and airtight building designs that do not include good ventilation. The list of possibilities is long.

If you believe you are suffering from sick building syndrome, it may be helpful to keep a journal in which you track your symptoms relative to the time spent in the building. If the problem building is your home, you can eliminate some or all of the toxins as described in this chapter. If the building is your place of work, you can speak to your employer about the problem and/or register a complaint with your local department of health. If you live in an apartment in the building, see if your neighbors are having similar problems and, if necessary, organize a protest. If the problem continues, you may have to find another place to live or work. It is often difficult to pinpoint the problem and remove the source.

The truth is that there is no one easy solution to the problems caused by a sick building. However, once you realize that a building is making you ill, you need to take action both for your own health and for the well-being of your family, neighbors, or coworkers.

Before the 1980s, asbestos was used in almost every public and commercial building as well as in ships. Although the link between exposure to asbestos, cancer, and various other diseases has been known since the 1930s, for many years, little was done to restrict its use. It wasn't until 1986 that the Environmental Protection Agency (EPA) required schools to remove any building materials containing asbestos. Although sixty-seven countries around the world have banned the use of asbestos, the United States has not. Instead, it relies on manufactures to work within suggested federal and state governmental guidelines. Although asbestos is no longer mined in the United States and its use has declined significantly, American industry still legally imports, uses, and sells both raw asbestos and products made with it.

If your house or apartment was built before 1980, you may have asbestos present, particularly in insulation materials covering hot water and steam pipes; in home siding shingles; and in floor and ceiling tiles. Asbestos can cause severe breathing problems, lung cancer, and mesothelioma, a type of cancer that occurs in the thin layer of tissue that covers the majority of your internal organs (mesothelium). If you have any construction going on in your home that exposes the insides of walls, floors, or ceilings, you need to ask your contractor to determine if there is asbestos present. If there is, you will need to hire specially trained experts to remove and dispose of it safely. This is not a job for an amateur. If your house is newer, it is unlikely that you have asbestos present. However, since the US has not banned the use of asbestos, it can still be found in many products, from tools to cookware to appliances.

Asbestos becomes more hazardous when it begins to crumble, is damaged, or is in a state of disrepair. Unfortunately, hiring a professional to remove asbestos from a home or office is not cheap, and for many, it is unaffordable. If you believe the building you are in contains exposed asbestos material, you should contact your local board of health to report it. However, for most of us, looking for another place to live or work may be a more realistic option. While I understand that this may not be an easy decision, it should be seriously considered in light of what could happen to you and your family.

Lead

Another deadly environmental contaminant is the toxic heavy metal lead. Lead poisoning occurs when too much of this substance gets into the body through the skin or from breathing, eating, or drinking. Lead is toxic to everyone, but is particularly harmful to unborn babies and young children, who can absorb lead more easily than older kids and adults. In children, lead poisoning can affect mental and physical development and cause numerous health issues. In adults, it can produce high blood pressure, body pain, mood disorders, miscarriages, and more.

Lead can contaminate food, water, soil, and the air we breathe. Remember that although some uses of lead—in paint and toys, for instance—have been banned in the United States, this toxic metal is still found in older products made in the US. Also, lead is still used in other countries, such as China. Although only small amounts may be found in certain products, such as cosmetics or some dishes, lead builds up in the body over time. Here are some common places where lead may be hiding.

- Lead paint, peeling, chipping on or in houses built *before* 1978. (Note that children may eat or suck on lead paint chips because they taste sweet.)

- Lead dust resulting from the sanding or scraping of houses built before 1978.

- Lead water pipes, which allow lead to leach into household water.

- Contaminated soil near an old gas station or near lead mining/ processing plants.

- Food or juice stored in lead-glazed food containers from other countries, such as China.

- Children's toys manufactured outside the United States.

- Dishes, including pet dishes, manufactured outside the United States.

- Some imported jewelry and candles.

- Cosmetics.

- Cigarettes.

If you have lead paint in your home, do not attempt to remove it yourself. Hire experts who have experience in removing lead from buildings. Do not let your children or pets remain in your home while the renovations are going on. If you live in a rented house or apartment, demand that your landlord pay for any needed renovations.

How do you know if you or your child has high lead levels? A simple blood test can measure the amount of lead in their body. Keep in mind that there is no safe blood level for lead, but a measure of 5 mcg/dL or more of lead suggests that there may be a problem that requires monitoring. There are drugs available that can help remove lead from the body.

Your local health department can offer guidance for testing paint, water, soil, and other sources of lead contamination. Most inspectors will come out to your home, perform lead inspection tests, and advise you on a course of action. Before they come, ask if there is a charge. For more information about lead poisoning in children and adults, see page 283 of the Resources section.

Mold

Mold is a serious biological pollutant. It can grow in damp basements, wet drywall and carpets, and near water leaks. It can appear as unwanted patches of black, brown, and green fuzzy growths. Some molds release poisonous mold gasses called mycotoxins—also known as mold VOC (volatile organic compounds), or MVOCs. When these gases are inhaled, they can cause a number of respiratory problems, including coughs, wheezing, nose and throat irritations, and asthma-like symptoms. Over time, mold can cause serious harm, mainly to the lungs. In addition, some people are severely allergic to even nontoxic molds.

ASTHMA AND POLLUTION

Asthma is a respiratory condition in which the bronchi (branches) of the lungs spasm, making it hard to breath. It affects both children and adults. Many different factors can trigger an asthmatic attack, including stress, infection, exercise, ozone, mold and other potential allergens, and VOCs (discussed on page 190). The body's inflammatory response causes the airways to swell, narrowing the airways and reducing the flow of air. Breathing problems may be mild to life-threatening.

The burden of asthma in the United States falls disproportionately on Black, Hispanic, and Native American people. These groups have the highest asthma rates, deaths, and hospitalizations. Although genetics play a role in asthma, the triggers are usually offending substances in the environment.

Asthma is a small portion of the overall healthcare problems seen in the underserved communities of the United States. It reflects the high frequency of disease in a population, and the marginalization of the care received. Many of the issues addressed in this book come together in this singular disease in communities of color, but are a true reflection of broader health and healthcare issues in America. In a recent report issued jointly by the Asthma and Allergy Foundation of America and the National Pharmaceutical Council, it was stated "that 40 percent of the risk of asthma in minority children is attributable to exposure to residential allergens that could be reduced, if not eliminated." With the help of your doctor, you must search for the triggers described in this chapter and eliminate them if possible.

If a basement, tenement building, home, or apartment has that old musty odor, it's most likely mold. Also, be aware that mold does not always have a strong odor, nor is it always visible. You may see a great deal of mold, a few spots of mold, or none at all. Molds like damp, dark, hidden spaces, and can grow above ceiling tiles, behind walls, in ductwork, or underneath carpet.

If you see mold and know that it isn't a dangerous form, you can try to remove it yourself. (See page 284 in the Resources section for websites that provide removal tips.) But if you only suspect that mold is growing in your home but can't find it, or if the mold is making you and your family sick, call in professionals to find and eliminate the problem. When a professional team arrives at your home to remove mold, they wear protective suits and hoods. This is an indication of how serious mold can be. In addition to removing the mold, the team can determine what kind of mold it is.

Plastics

Many plastics (but not all) contain a group of toxic chemicals known as *phthalates*, which make plastics more flexible and harder to break. They are released as fumes and dust particles as the plastic products age, when they are exposed to heat, or as they come into contact with food and water. Unfortunately, phthalates are everywhere—in plastic bags, garden hoses, inflatable recreational toys, intravenous tubing, shower curtains, kitchen utensils, baby products, personal-care products such as soaps and shampoos, and more. They are polluting our bodies, and just as bad, they are polluting the oceans and waterways with junk that will not likely disintegrate any time this century.

Phthalates are the most commonly found manmade chemicals in the environment. And yes, these chemicals are even found in our blood, our breast milk, and our urine. Once they enter the body, they break down into other harmful chemicals.

You won't believe the number of major public health concerns that are related to phthalates. These include asthma, attention-deficit hyperactivity disorder (ADHD), autism, low IQ, breast cancer, obesity, type 2 diabetes, male fertility issues—and these are just the ones that have been studied.

This problem is not particular to African Americans. This is a world-wide problem affecting everyone. Nevertheless, with all the other toxins that face us, phthalates are unneeded pollutants with devastating consequences. It's impossible to completely avoid phthalates, but to minimize exposure, avoid vinyl toys, perfumed shampoos and lotions (choose fragrance-free personal-care products whenever possible), and packaged and processed foods. Studies have shown that children get exposed to the highest concentration of these chemicals by common packaged foods—probably because phthalates are present both in the food and in the packaging, which transfers more phthalates to the food. Since these chemicals can have serious effects on infants and children, it's important to protect your kids as much as possible.

Volatile Organic Compounds (VOC)

The most common contaminants of indoor spaces are VOCs, or *volatile organic compounds*, which are emitted as gases from certain solids or liquids. VOCs are the invisible chemicals we smell when we bring paint products, building supplies, and even new furniture into our homes. The evaporation process is referred to as "off-gassing," and it can last long after the new paint smell is gone—potentially, for several years. Some of the more familiar chemicals that emit VOCs include benzene, ethanol, formaldehyde, and toluene.

VOCs can often be found in the following products:

- Aerosol sprays
- Air fresheners
- Carpets
- Cleansers and disinfectants
- Dry-cleaned clothing
- Hobby supplies
- Moth repellents
- Paints, paint strippers, and other solvents
- Pesticides
- Wood preservatives
- Stored fuels and automotive products

The ability of VOCs to cause health effects varies greatly from those with no known health effects to those that are highly toxic. And as with other pollutants, the extent and nature of the health problem depends on many factors, including level of exposure and length of time exposed. Following are some of the symptoms associated with exposure to VOCs:

- Allergic skin reaction
- Dizziness

- Eye irritation
- Fatigue
- Headache
- Nausea

- Nose and throat discomfort
- Nose bleeds
- Respiratory tract irritation
- Vomiting

To avoid the problems caused by VOCs, do what you can to buy products that don't contain these chemicals. In some cases, this is fairly easy. Many house paints, for instance, now state that they have low or no VOCs. When buying cleaners, look for organic products made with nontoxic ingredients. If you do have to use a

YOUR CARPET MAY BE MAKING YOU SICK

Did you know even your carpet, both new and old, gives off toxic fumes—the VOCs discussed on page 190? You know the smell of a new carpet? I actually like that smell because it makes me think of something new and clean. Unfortunately, it's toxic because it contains chemicals such as formaldehyde, xylene, benzene, toluene, 4-phenylcyclohexene (4-PCH), and styrene—some of the same chemicals discussed in the section above. The fact is that new carpets can off-gas VOCs for five to fifteen years or more after installation. Just like other household products that contain these chemicals, toxin-laden carpets can cause a variety of symptoms, and can be especially harmful to family members who have asthma and other respiratory disorders.

Due to the health problems caused by toxic carpets in both homes and workplaces, the Carpet and Rug Institute now uses a "Green Label" to help you identify the lowest emitting carpets. Be aware that VOCs are emitted not only by the carpet but also by the adhesives and padding installed with the carpet. So for the safety of yourself and your family, it makes sense to make sure that your new floor covering and all the products associated with it have the Green Label.

product that contains toxic chemicals, try to work in a well-ventilated area and wear a respirator mask. For more information on buying safer products, see page 283 of the Resources section.

POLLUTION IN SCHOOLS

While most of us spend a large portion of our time at home, children spend hundreds of hours each year in school, and children are especially vulnerable to the health and developmental impacts of environmental toxins. Studies have shown that poor indoor air quality in schools is linked to decreased concentration and poor test results while also adding to asthma attacks, headaches, fatigue, nausea, and rashes.

In a 2018 article in the journal *Environmental Research*, scientists studied exposures to neurotoxins—harmful chemicals that affect the nervous system—in the areas around roughly 85,000 public schools. Black and poor children were far more likely to attend schools in areas polluted by neurotoxins. The scientists reported that urban areas were more likely polluted than rural school, and that children in pre-kindergarten had the highest risks. More than a quarter of Black children attended school in areas with the *worst* pollution. The author, Dr. Sara Grineski, stated, "This could well be impacting an entire generation of our society."

What about your child's school? Consider the following:

- If your child's school is old and has leaky roofs that cause ceilings, walls, or floors to be moist or wet, molds may be present that are giving off toxic fumes. This can make the children (and the teacher) sick.

- If lead paint is peeling off the walls or lead dust is in the air because of renovations, the lead particles can poison the children. If asbestos is present in the air, that can cause severe respiratory symptoms.

- If your child's school is next to freeways and downtown traffic, exhaust fumes can seep into the school, harming the children. VOCs in the air around the school can also seep in.

- If your child's school has rodents or roaches, pesticides may be used by school authorities to kill them. Even if these sprays are applied at night, the toxic fumes will still be present the next day.

- Perfumes and aftershave fragrances used by teachers and the staff may also be present. Room fresheners may make the class-room smell better but cause some students to feel sick.

- New schools and recently renovated schools could be polluted by new flooring or carpets, plastics, paints, and cabinets that are giving off toxic gases.

What can you do if you suspect your child's school is contaminated? Talk to other parents and encourage them to fight for their children, too. Perhaps as a group, you can meet with the teachers and principal. If you don't feel you are making any progress, make an appointment with one or more members of the school board. Then contact your congressman and senators. Call the local news-paper and TV stations to express your concerns. Make your voices heard! You may have more power than you realized.

IMPROVING INDOOR AIR QUALITY

As you have learned, your home, your office, and your child's school can be a trap for noxious fumes and particulates. According to the Environmental Protection Agency, improving indoor air quality requires four steps:

Eliminate the Source

As we have discussed throughout this chapter, air pollution inside a home, office, or school can come from a number of sources, ranging from mold to paint to carpets and other furnish-ings. Some sources may be in plain sight, while others may be less obvious. By identifying and removing them, you can create a safer environment for yourself, your family, and/or your coworkers or staff. In some cases, you may not be able to eliminate the problem on your own. In such a case, you can either call in professional help or let your state or local department of health know about the problem.

Improve Ventilation

According to the EPA, improving ventilation is the most effective means of improving clean air at home. While heating, ventilation, and air conditioning (HVAC) systems may make you comfortable, they do not do a good job of exchanging air in your home.

Improving ventilation is relatively simple. Indoor air quality is a function of the amount of fresh air moving throughout the building. When the air isn't moving, a greater amount of toxic gases, such as VOCs, float around your home. This may cause increased headaches, shortness of breath, and asthma attacks. The EPA recommends that when weather allows, you open windows and doors, operate window or attic fans, or run a window air conditioner with the vent control open. Kitchen and bathroom fans that exhaust outdoors remove contaminants directly from the room where the fan is located.

Beside pollution issues in your home, there may also be air pollution at your workplace. This too should be addressed, especially if you notice you are becoming ill at work. No doubt, at the workplace, unless you are the owner or manager, this may prove to be a challenge. However, keep in mind that they are likely to be breathing in the same air, and may wind up having the same health issues.

Use Air Purifiers

Air purifiers are generally not designed to remove harmful fumes, but instead, tiny particles. This includes ash, dirt, dust, pollen, and smoke. The effectiveness of an air cleaner depends on how well it collects pollutants from indoor air and how much air it draws through the cleaning or filtering element. Normally, air filtration units come with a list of the particles they are designed to remove from your environment. Be sure to keep the filters clean and to replace them as necessary.

Grow Plants That Cleanse the Air

While air purifiers can be expensive, plants generally are inexpensive and often require minimal care. In their search for methods to clean the air in space stations, NASA—the National Aeronautics and Space Administration—found that plants can "scrub" the air of toxic gases, including VOC-emitting substances such as benzene and formaldehyde. In addition, plants absorb the carbon dioxide in the air and release fresh oxygen. This is an easy and decorative way of cleaning the air in your home along with removing pollutants.

Plants that reduce indoor pollution include Dwarf Date Palm, Boston Fern, Kimberley Queen Fern, Spider Plants, Chinese Evergreen, Bamboo Palm, Weeping Fig, Devil's Ivy, Flamingo Lily, and Lily Turf. NASA found that for every 100 square feet in your home, you need one plant. Some of these plants, such as spider plants, are often easily available in nurseries and even home goods stores. To learn more about plants that can improve air quality, see page 282 of the Resources section.

DETOXIFICATION

At the start of this chapter, we said that there are two environments with which we should be concerned. The first is the *external environment*—the objects, chemicals, and compounds we're exposed to daily. This is the environment we've discussed so far in this chapter. The second is the *internal environment*—everything inside the body. As you know, the external environment can greatly impact the internal environment. The term *toxic load* is used to refer to the accumulation of toxins and chemicals in our bodies that come from a variety of sources, including the air we breathe, the food we eat, the water we drink, and the personal care and house products we use. When our toxic load increases, we can get sick and experience the symptoms described in this chapter, such as headache, fatigue, and more serious health disorders. To make matters worse, none of us knows how bad our toxic load really is. That's why the rest of this chapter explores ways in which you can detoxify your body.

Detoxification is the process of removing or cleansing toxic substances from your body. The good news is that there are a number of ways to detox the body naturally, without invasive treatments. I want to make clear that since you don't how much toxic material has accumulated in your body, there will be no scientific way to measure the effectiveness of your detoxification efforts. The best indicator will be how you feel afterwards.

Detoxifying Through Water Intake and Exercise

A healthy human body is always detoxifying itself. It uses the liver, kidneys (urine), bowels (stool), skin (sweat), and respiratory system to identify and eliminate waste products and toxins. The problem is that between the unhealthy foods we often eat and the unhealthy environments in which we live, the body often is flooded with more harmful substances than it can easily handle. That's why it's important to give it some help.

If you want to work in tune with your body, all you have to do are two things: drink lots of water and sweat as much as you can through exercise. Ideally, men need to drink between 15 to 18 cups of water, and woman, between 11 to 13 cups—in general, between three and four quarts of water a day. Of course, these requirements also depend on your height and weight, on the amount of exercise you do, and on any health conditions you have. It's a good idea to discuss your ideal water intake with your doctor. Believe it or not, it is possible to drink too much water.

A healthy exercise routine will help your body eliminate toxins through sweat. It will also have an impact on the amount of water you drink. If you do a twenty-minute workout each day and you see yourself sweating more, drink more water. If you choose to do a more vigorous workout, take in more water. It shouldn't cost you anything, and you will be eliminating lots of unwanted substances from your body. If you want to take it a step further, you can go into a hot tub or sauna. For information on healthy exercise, turn to page 39. If you have any health conditions, speak to your healthcare provider before introducing exercise to your life.

Choosing Non-Toxic Foods

The majority of produce grown commercially contains small amounts of herbicides and pesticides. Meat products contain hormones and antibiotics, while fish contains whatever pollutants happen to be in the water, but can be especially high in mercury, a heavy metal. In fact, commercial foods are one of our most serious sources of toxicity.

To decrease your toxic load (discussed on page 195), find stores that offer organic meat and poultry as well as at least some organic fruits, vegetables, and canned and frozen foods. Yes, these products are more expensive, but they are cheaper than visits to the doctor. Keep in mind that some produce that's grown conventionally contains more pesticides than others, so if you want to be careful with your money, you can buy organic versions of produce that typically has high pesticide residue, like apples and strawberries; but choose less expensive conventional produce when buying produce that typically has less pesticide residue, such as onions and corn. To help guide you, every year, the Environmental Working Group (EWG) provides a list of the Dirty Dozen (produce with the most pesticides) and the Clean Fifteen (produce that's low in pesticides). (See page 285 of the Resources list for the website.) The EWG will also guide you to seafood that's low in mercury.

Detoxifying Through Fasting

In Chapter 9, we discussed how fasting provides a range of benefits, including better weight control, better blood sugar control, and detoxification. When you eat throughout the day, your digestive system, liver, and kidneys are continuously working to absorb nutrients and flush toxins out of your body. When you fast, the body gets a break from digestion and can spend more time on detoxification.

I recommend intermittent fasting, which has three variations. Turn to page 173 of Chapter 9 to learn about the variations and choose the method that's right for you. Just remember that while intermittent fasting includes times when you don't eat food, you should *never* eliminate fluids during your fasts. Your body needs water to function, and as you learned earlier in this chapter, water is vital for detoxifying your body.

CONCLUSION

Unfortunately, the majority of African Americans live in a polluted environment that contributes to health disorders. I understand that not every brother or sister lives in a highly polluted town or city, but all too many of us do. Because most environmental toxins are hidden from sight, we don't think about them, and we allow them to make us and our children sick. While we can take steps to improve our homes, there is little we can to do clean up the bigger picture—unless we make it a priority.

Those in political power and in industry know that as a community, we have been relatively silent on the issue of the environment. While industries are sometimes forced by the government to make changes, they have not made changes to improve the health of Black communities. Now that you know how environmental pollution can affect your well-being, it's vital to use your pocketbook and your voice to demand that actions be taken.

When we saw George Floyd with a knee on his neck crying out "I can't breathe," it started a movement. When you hear a Black child with asthma cry "I can't breathe," it's a sign that we must initiate a movement to eliminate pollution from our neighborhoods. Just as being silent about racism doesn't help our cause, neither will accepting the toxic environment we live in. If knowledge is power, you now have the power to make the world a cleaner, healthier place for you and your family.

11

Sickle Cell Disease

"No matter how big a nation is, it is no stronger than its weakest people, and as long as you keep a person down, some part of you has to be down there to hold him down, so it means you cannot soar as you might otherwise."
—MARIAN ANDERSON

There are few diseases that focus on just a few groups of people. *Sickle cell disease (SCD)*, commonly called sickle cell anemia, is one of them. It is an inherited disease, not a contagious one like the flu. For the Black and Hispanic communities, hearing that you have SCD is almost as bad as being told you have cancer. This disease affects one out of 16,300 Hispanic Americans. However, for every African-American child born, that number is one out of every 365. Because this is a relatively common disease in our community, it is important to understand what this disease is, how it affects those who have it, and how it can be managed.

A few years ago, there was very little anyone could do to help people suffering from SCD. Today, however, medical research has made important discoveries that may offer a path to a healthier life for many suffering from this disease. In this chapter, we will answer some of the most common questions you may have about sickle cell disease.

WHAT IS SICKLE CELL DISEASE?

Sickle cell disease is a genetic-based disease of the blood that affects the red blood cells. Red blood cells (RBCs) are the key to life because they deliver oxygen throughout the body while removing the waste product carbon dioxide so it can be exhaled. Microscopic round discs that are concave on both sides, RBCs contain a compound known as *hemoglobin*, which is the special protein that carries the oxygen. Because the cells are round but flexible, they are able to bend and slide through the extremely tiny blood vessels called capillaries. In SCD, however, RBCs become misshapen. Instead of being concave disks, they become sickle or crescent shaped and much less flexible. (See Figure 11.1.) Therefore, they not only carry less oxygen but also pass through capillaries with difficulty and sometimes get stuck, blocking the blood vessel. This prevents other cells from getting through and causes clumping and a decrease in blood flow, preventing sufficient oxygen and nutrients from being delivered to the body's tissues.

HOW IS SCD INHERITED?

SCD is caused by an abnormal gene—a unit of heredity—that is passed by *both* parents to their child. (If only one parent has

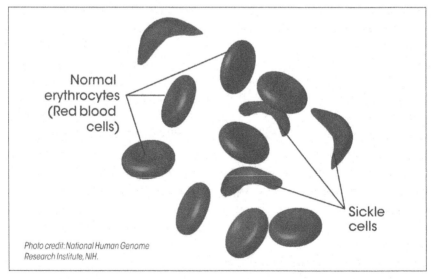

Normal
erythrocytes
(Red blood
cells)

Sickle
cells

Photo credit: National Human Genome
Research Institute, NIH.

Figure 11.1. Normal Red Blood Cells Next to Sickle Blood Cells.

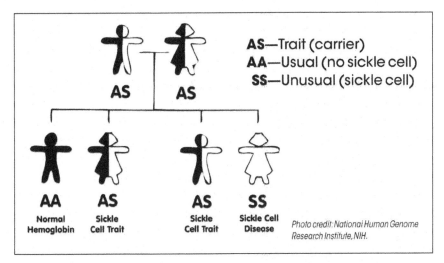

AS—Trait (carrier)
AA—Usual (no sickle cell)
SS—Unusual (sickle cell)

AS   AS

AA   AS   AS   SS

Normal   Sickle   Sickle   Sickle Cell
Hemoglobin Cell Trait   Cell Trait Disease   Photo credit: National Human Genome
                                                      Research Institute, NIH.

Figure 11.2. How Sickle Cell Disease Is Inherited from
Two Parents with the Sickle Cell Trait.

the bad gene, the child gets the *SC trait*, which usually causes no symptoms.) Note that in Figure 11.2, the two parents with sickle cell traits each have one good gene (A) and one bad gene (S). By chance, if they had four children, they could have one child with a *normal hemoglobin gene* (AA), two with the *sickle cell trait* (AS), and one child with *sickle cell disease* (SS).

THE DIFFERENT TYPES OF SCD

Sickle cell disease is an umbrella term for several forms of SCD. The various types are listed below.

- **HEMOGLOBIN SS DISEASE.** This is the most common type of SCD, accounting for 65 percent of all childhood cases. This condition occurs when two bad sickle cell genes are inherited from both parents. It is the most severe form of SCD and causes a high rate of the worst symptoms.

- **HEMOGLOBIN SC.** This form of sickle cell disease accounts for 25 percent of all SCD cases in children. The baby receives one sickle cell gene and another abnormal hemoglobin gene known as C.

The onset of symptoms is often delayed to later childhood, and while symptoms are similar to those of hemoglobin SS disease, they are usually less frequent and severe.

- **HEMOGLOBIN S-BETA-THALASSEMIA.** This accounts for about 10 percent of SCD cases. The child inherits one bad sickle cell gene and another defective hemoglobin (beta-thalassemia), in which some normal hemoglobin is produced. In such cases, the individual may have milder symptoms than someone with SCD.

- **HEMOGLOBIN SD, HEMOGLOBIN SE, AND HEMOGLOBIN SO.** These three type of SCD are very rare, and normally do not result in severe symptoms.

- **SICKLE CELL TRAIT.** This occurs when a person inherits an abnormal gene from one parent, but not both. This may result in a few symptoms or no symptoms at all. However, people with the affected gene can pass it on to their children.

Each of these disorders can be identified through testing during pregnancy, at birth, and throughout a person's life.

TESTING FOR SICKLE CELL DISEASE

Simple tests can detect the defective form of hemoglobin that underlies sickle cell anemia. If sickle cell disease is present in your family, ask that during a pregnancy, a sample of the amniotic fluid surrounding the fetus be tested for the gene abnormality. If the fetus has SCD, you may be referred to a hematologist, who specializes in blood disorders and can help you and your baby after birth.

After birth, all newborn infants in every state in the United States are required by law to be screened for potential developmental, genetic, and metabolic disorders. This includes SCD. Therefore, parents will know right from birth whether or not their infant has the disorder. If your child was not born in a hospital, ask your doctor to perform this critical screening test.

In young children and babies, the blood sample is usually collected from a finger or heel. In adults, blood is drawn from a vein in the arm. If you or your child has sickle cell anemia, your doctor may suggest additional tests to check for possible complications of the disease.

SYMPTOMS AND COMPLICATIONS OF SICKLE CELL ANEMIA

The symptoms and complications associated with SCD can vary according to age—newborns can experience symptoms different from those of older individuals—and according to the individual with the disorder. Virtually all of the major symptoms of the disease are the result of the abnormally shaped red blood cells blocking the flow of blood. The tissues with impaired circulation suffer damage from lack of oxygen, potentially causing severe disability and episodes of severe pain.

SCD Symptoms in Newborns

Most babies with SCD will start exhibiting symptoms within the first year of life. The symptoms can include extreme fussiness; swelling, redness, and tenderness of the hands and feet; and a yellowing of the skin, eyes, and mouth caused by jaundice.

In addition, associated symptoms can include fever, coughing, breathing problems, pain in the bones, fatigue, and headaches. If the baby is always crying or cries when you touch him in areas of the body that appear red for no reason, you should immediately contact your physician.

Anemia

Anemia is a condition marked by a deficiency of healthy red blood cells or of hemoglobin, the protein that carries oxygen in the blood. This results in pale, flat colored skin (meaning that the skin looks drained) and chronic fatigue. Tests for anemia include a complete blood count to see if you have a lower red blood cell count. Often, an *H and H test* is perform to measure the *hematocrit,* or the proportion of red blood cells in the blood, as well as the amount of hemoglobin in the blood. Chronic anemia from infancy and childhood often delays puberty and slows growth.

Infections

"Sicklers"—people with SCD—are more susceptible to infection than people who don't have this disorder. SCD often damages the spleen by blocking the blood vessels that lead out of the organ. The spleen plays an important role in the immune system by producing the white blood cells (WBCs), called lymphocytes, that fight off infections. If the spleen is unable to produce sufficient WBCs, the person with SCD becomes vulnerable to foreign bacteria, viruses, and other harmful microbes. That's why infants and children with SCD are given preventive antibiotics and vaccinations for several different childhood diseases. (See page 207 for more information on these preventive measures.) With recurring damage to the spleen caused by blood vessel blockage, some people with SCD eventually require the removal of the spleen through a procedure called a splenectomy.

Vision Problems

Just as sickle cells can block the capillaries in other portions of the body, they can cause blockage of blood vessels in the retina and

---

GETTING HELP IN AN EMERGENCY ROOM

One of the worst things about SCD is that you may be denied pain relief in an emergency room because you are Black. Doctors and nurses often don't understand SCD and the kind of intense pain it can cause. Ask your doctor to prepare a letter you can carry with you about sickle cell anemia, its effects, and the need for narcotic pain relief. A copy of your lab results should be included. When and if you have to go to an emergency room, you can hand the information to the doctor in charge of your case and ask that he or she contact your physician if necessary.

choroid, causing a thinning of the retina and abnormal blood vessel growth. This disorder, called *sickle cell retinopathy*, affects roughly 30 to 40 percent of patients with SCD by age twenty. Symptoms can include blind spots, the sudden onset of floaters or blurred vision, flashes of light, and the loss of side vision.

Pain

The lack of adequate oxygen associated with sickle cell disease causes pain as cells begin dying and become damaged. This remains the single greatest problem of SCD patients—constant or recurrent acute and chronic pain. Given that pain is the number-one reason for SCD patients to go to the hospital, it is important to state that these patients often experience racial bias every time they go for treatment. Specifically, studies reveal that a substantial number of white laypeople, medical students, and residents do not view and treat pain in Black people as they view and treat pain in White people.

The pain these patients experience is usually in their chest, abdomen, joints, and bones. It may last for a few hours or even weeks. The cruelty occurs because when an SCD person comes to the hospital, it's almost never for the first time, so their medical records are available. Nevertheless, pain medications are often withheld because the hospital staff believes that the patients are there "for drug-seeking purposes." The fact is that they are! They have sickle cell disease and are in crisis!

A SCD crisis—medically called a *vaso-occlusive crisis*—occurs when sickled cells start clumping together and block capillaries. Almost anything can set off the crisis—an infection, fatigue, dehydration, and other factors. Once clumps form, these cells are unable to pass through the capillaries, creating a backlog on one side and ischemia (the lack of blood flow) on the other. Where there's ischemia, there's also a partial or total lack of oxygen and essential nutrients going to organs. This can become critical, causing damage to bones, a stroke, delayed growth, anemia, and even death.

STANDARD TREATMENTS FOR SICKLE CELL DISEASE

There are several treatments available for the person with sickle cell anemia. Pain relief is especially important, but treatments are also available to prevent infection and to infuse the blood with normal red blood cells.

Pain Relief and the Prevention of Vaso-Occlusive Crises

As you've already learned, pain is the symptom that most often brings the person with SCD to a hospital for help. The following medications can be used to treat the pain of sickle cell disease and to prevent the medical crises most often responsible for sickle cell-related pain.

- *Crizanlizumab (Adakveo)* is a monoclonal antibody medication used to prevent vaso-occlusive crisis in patients with sickle cell anemia. Given intravenously, it can cause side effects, including nausea, joint pain, back pain, and fever.

- *Hydroxyurea (Droia, Siklos)* is in a class of medications called anti-metabolites. It treats sickle cell anemia by helping to prevent the formation of sickle-shaped red blood cells. Although it reduces the frequency of painful crises and blood transfusions, it can also increase the susceptibility to infection.

- *L-glutamine* is a natural amino acid. Oral therapy with phar-maceutical-grade L-glutamine has been medically approved to reduce the frequency of sick cell-related pain.

- *Narcotics* are a group of drugs now called opioids. Your doctor might prescribe narcotics to help relieve pain during sickle cell pain crises. Of course, when you talk about narcotics, there's always the possibility of addiction. See the inset on page 208 for more about this issue.

- *Voxelotor (Oxbryta)* improves anemia by inhibiting red blood cell sickling. Through this mechanism, it increases oxygen saturation and reduces the need for hospital admission due to episodes of vaso-occlusive crisis pain. Potential side effects of treatment with this medication include headache, stomach pain, nausea, fatigue, and fever.

Preventing Infections

As we already discussed, because sickle cell disease damages the spleen—which normally plays an important part in the immune response—people with SCD have an increased risk of developing certain infections, including pneumonia, blood stream and bone infections, and meningitis. The following medications are often used to prevent such infections.

- *Penicillin* is often given to children between the ages of two months and five years of age to prevent infections before they start. Add yogurt and probiotics to your child's diet to replace the gut bacteria killed by the penicillin. (Turn to page 22 to learn about probiotic foods and supplements.)

- *Vaccinations* can prevent many of the more serious infections. Talk to your doctor about the shots that you or your young child should receive, including vaccinations for hepatitis A and B; measles, mumps, and rubella (German measles); chickenpox; rotavirus, Haemophilus influenzae, tetanus, diphtheria, and pertussis; and poliovirus. Each year, your doctor may recommend shots for pneumococcal bacteria, which causes pneumonia and other infections; the flu; and meningococcus, which causes meningitis.

Blood Transfusions

Transfusions are designed to improve the blood by adding to the number of healthy red blood cells.

- **TRANSFUSIONS.** Red blood cells from a blood donor may be given to increase the number of normal red blood cells. These transfusions help lessen the anemia and reduce the blood's viscosity (thickness), enabling it to flow more freely and thus preventing complications such as stroke and vaso-occlusive crisis. If you need transfusions frequently, your blood may contain excess

SICKLERS AND DRUG ADDICTION

In today's world, doctors and patients are worried about pre-scribing or receiving pain relieving narcotics, which are known to be potentially addictive. This issue was addressed at a National Institute of Health conference by sickle cell disease expert Wally Smith, MD, who stated, "Contrary to popular belief, most patients with sickle cell disease who are on opioid painkillers don't become addicts. It is these patients who are hurt by the well-meaning war on opioids. . . . But determining which patients will benefit the most remains a challenge." Smith also reported that the estimated prevalence of opioid addiction in the sickle cell population is about 10 percent, no more than the addiction rate found in other chronic pain populations.

If you or your child is receiving multiple prescriptions of nar-cotics for sickle cell-related pain, discuss this issue with your doctor.

iron, which can damage the heart, liver, and other organs. If this occurs, iron chelators—medicines that bind with iron—may be used to help remove the excess iron from your body.

PROMISING NEW TREATMENTS FOR SICKLE CELL DISEASE

Twenty-first-century medical technology has made several major breakthroughs in the treatment of SCD—bone marrow transplants and gene therapy. While these techniques are still being tested and refined, they show great promise in the treatment of SCD, and in some cases, can even eliminate the disease.

Bone Marrow (Stem Cell) Transplants

Bone marrow (stem cell) transplant is the only treatment available today that can cure sickle cell disease.

A *stem cell* is a special type of cell found in your bone marrow, the soft substance in the cavities of your bones that produces red blood cells. Stem cells are immature cells, meaning they can develop into many different kinds of cells—whatever your body needs. The goal of the transplant is to replace the individual's bone marrow with healthy bone marrow so that the person's body can start to produce normal hemoglobin.

For years, bone marrow transplants were performed only on children because of the risk associated with transplants in adults. High-dose chemotherapy is used to destroy all of a child's bone marrow to get rid of the defective gene. The marrow is then replaced with healthy stem cells from a donor—normally, a brother or sister who has closely matching bone marrow. Recipients must take drugs for months or even years to prevent the body from rejecting the donor's cells. These drugs can have serious side effects, so the child must be monitored carefully.

Now, new methods of performing bone marrow transplants are making it possible to successfully perform them in some adults. Between 2004 and 2013, thirty patients, ages 16 to 65, with severe SCD were studied by researchers at the National Institute of Health. The patients first took drugs to kill off *some* but not all of their marrow cells. They then had stem cell transplants with cells donated by a healthy brother or sister. The disease was reversed in some but not all of the patients. Still, the risks of stem cell transplant become greater as a person gets older and/or develops damage to major organs. For this reason, bone marrow transplants are not a treatment option for most adults with SCD.

If you are interested in bone marrow transplants, see if your community has a Medical School and Research Center. Call them to ask if they are doing stem cell transplants for sickle cell. If they are not, ask for the nearest center, or ask your doctor about these transplants. Some centers include the University of Michigan in Bethesda, Maryland; St Jude's Children's Research Hospital in Memphis, Tennessee; Texas Children's Hospital in Houston; and St. Louis Children's Hospital in Missouri.

Gene Therapy

Because SCD is a genetic disorder, you may be wondering if doctors can simply replace the bad gene with a normal one. *Gene therapy* is a promising technique that uses healthy genes to prevent or treat a disease. This can include replacing or inactivating a disease-causing gene or introducing a new or modified gene to help treat a disease.

In the treatment of sickle cell disease, a normal therapeutic gene for hemoglobin is donated to someone with sickle cell disease. The normal gene is injected into stem cells removed from a sickle cell patient and then returned to the patient, where the modified stem cells develop into normal red blood cells. Of course, it's more complicated than that, but the technique is being refined and tested, and the results seem promising. In one study, researchers at Boston Children's Hospital found that six patients who were treated with gene therapy and followed for up to twenty-nine months suffered fewer or none of the severe flare-ups that characterize SCD. Based on preliminary findings, researchers believe that in the near future, gene replacement therapy will enable the patients' bone marrow to produce normal red blood cells consistently.

THE LIFE EXPECTANCY OF PEOPLE WITH SCD

People with sickle cell disease have a reduced life expectancy, but life span varies widely from one person to another. While some people do not survive beyond infancy or early childhood, some can remain without symptoms for years. New treatments for the disease are improving both the quality of life and the life span. If SCD is well managed, people can survive beyond their fifties. As new technology is perfected, the prognosis will continue to improve.

WHAT YOU CAN DO AT HOME

At this time, doctors can offer limited help for the person with sickle cell disease. Most of their arsenal of weapons is geared toward alleviating the pain associated with SCD. Fortunately, you can do a great deal to help yourself remain as healthy as possible. Your greatest emphasis should be on getting the nutrients you need to keep your body strong and to prevent medical crises.

Adjust Your Diet

Patients with SCD have special dietary needs, requiring more calories and more micronutrients (vitamins and minerals) than people who do not have SCD. The Physicians Committee for Responsible Medicine has recommended that people with sickle cell disease consume a high-calorie, nutrient-dense diet. This means that the diet must be super-nutritious without fatty, sugary, or salty processed foods.

Your diet should emphasize fruits and vegetables paired with whole grains and proteins—eggs, fish, chicken, meat, beans, tofu, and nuts and seeds. Also get plenty of calcium-rich foods and beverages, such as milk, yogurt, and cheese. This will provide a greater proportion of essential nutrients than can be found in a typical Western diet, and can help prevent deficiencies that can increase the likelihood of disease. Finally, consume eight 8-ounce glasses of water each day so that you can prevent the dehydration that can trigger a crisis.

Take Supplements

As explained above, people with sickle cell disease require more vitamins, minerals, and other micronutrients than people who are not battling this disease. While a super-nutritious diet can help, it's usually helpful to enhance your nutrient intake by taking key supplements. To ensure you're buying the best supplements, see the guidelines that begin on page 258. Because you or your child has special needs due to SCD, it's important to talk to your healthcare provider before adding supplements to your daily regimen.

Multivitamins

Nutrients including vitamin A, vitamin B_6, vitamin C, vitamin E, magnesium, and zinc are typically low in the blood of sicklers. To make sure you're getting these important substances, take a good multivitamin-mineral tablet. Your healthcare provider can guide you to a supplement that is best for your specific needs.

Vitamin D

Vitamin D deficiency is also very common in sicklers—no surprise, since I'm talking about a Black population—and must be supplemented to help bones grow normally, decrease bone fractures, and improve muscle weakness. In one study, children and adolescents with SCD who had low vitamin D levels had more frequent and longer hospital stays and made more visits to the emergency room.

For most people, 2,000 IU to 5,000 IU per day of vitamin D_3 is beneficial. You can also ask your healthcare provider to test your vitamin D levels and prescribe a dosage based on your test results. Make sure that your physician orders the 25-OH vitamin D test, as this will give you the best indication of your vitamin D body stores.

Omega-3 Fatty Acids

Omega-3 fatty acids have also been found to be low in people with SCD. Supplements of EPA and DHA can increase the fluidity of red blood cells, allowing them to slip more easily through capillaries. In a study from Sudan, researchers gave a group of sicklers an EPA and DHA fatty acid supplement and another group a placebo. Those who received the fatty acids had less anemia, needed fewer transfusions, and had fewer episodes of pain than those in the placebo group.

You can, of course, increase your omega-3s by eating more fatty fish, such as anchovies, herring, salmon, and mackerel, which are rich in this nutrient. But because it's hard to get all the omega-3s that you need to help you manage your SCD, I also suggest taking supplements. Between 1,000 and 2,000 mg per day of omega-3 fatty acids should help improve your condition so that you experience fewer symptom.

Folic Acid

Bone marrow needs folic acid (vitamin B_9) to make new red blood cells. Because of the high red blood cell turnover in people with

SCD, folate stores are often depleted. For this reason, children and adults with SCD often take 1 mg of folic acid orally every day to reduce the symptoms of anemia. Especially if you are treating a child, you should check with your doctor about the proper folic acid dosage.

Other Helpful Advice

In addition to improving your nutrient intake, you can take other steps to maintain the best possible health and avoid painful medical crises.

- Take your prescribed medication, including pain drugs, exactly as directed by your doctor.

- Dress warmly in cold weather. Exposure to cold air, wind, and water can cause a painful event by constricting the blood vessels in exposed areas of the body, causing the red blood cells to stick together. Dress in layers to avoid sudden temperature changes, and when possible, avoid situations in which you might become cold.

- Exercise with care. If you exercise strenuously, rest when you feel tired, and drink plenty of fluids to prevent dehydration. Dehydration and reduced oxygen levels can cause red blood cells to clump.

- Drink plenty of fluids, particularly during hot weather. As already explained, dehydration increases the risk of a sickle cell crisis.

- Avoid alcohol and smoking. Alcohol can cause you to become dehydrated, and smoking can trigger a serious lung condition called acute chest syndrome.

CONCLUSION

In the future, bone marrow transplants and gene therapy may make it possible for people born with sickle cell disease to live normal lives with normal life spans. In the meantime, there is a great deal you can do to manage your or your child's SCD, from eating a nutrient-rich diet to avoiding alcohol and smoking. Even dressing properly in cold or changeable weather can help you avoid painful crises and hospitalizations.

As a parent of a child with SCD or as a SCD patient, you know it's difficult to live with this disease. But it's important to also recognize that in a relatively short time, SCD may become a disease of the past.

12

Oral Health*

*"Every time you smile at someone, it is an action
of love, a gift to that person, a beautiful thing."*
—MOTHER TERESA

I n the first chapter, we discussed the importance of the gut-
microbiome-brain connection (GMB) for your health. Your gut
actually starts with your mouth. When you visit your physician,
the first thing he or she does is to look into your eyes, ears, and
mouth. If your mouth is not healthy, there is a good chance that
your body is also not healthy. This is because in addition to showing gum disease and tooth decay, your mouth can show signs of
many other conditions. It tells a story without your saying one
word. If you are missing certain foods in your diet or you have a
vitamin deficiency, the lack of proper nutrition may be abundantly
clear in your mouth. In fact, poor eating and living habits are a
major contributor to the many oral diseases and disparities that
cause suffering in the African-American community.

In this chapter, you will learn about common dental and oral
problems and explore how poor dental health affects our overall
health—how, amazingly, it impacts even the heart, blood sugar levels, blood pressure, and more. Toward the end of the chapter, we
will examine the difficulty that Black Americans have in finding
good affordable healthcare. But don't despair. You will learn the

---

* Contributed by Sonya Dunbar, RDH, MHA.

many steps you can take to promote better oral health, and you will find ways you may not have known about to obtain access to dental care.

TOOTH DECAY AND LOSS

When most people think about oral problems, they think about tooth decay and loss. In fact, cavities and tooth decay are among the world's most common health problems—especially in children, teenagers, and older adults. And, as you will learn later in the chapter, these problems are even worse in the Black community.

Preventive dental visits normally should take place once or—even better—twice a year. At these visits, the teeth are cleaned of plaque and tartar (which are discussed below), and the dentist checks for signs of tooth decay or gum disease. X-rays may also be taken. Sadly, many minority families are unaware of this fact, fail to make the necessary appointments, or cannot afford the visits. In the absence of these visits, tooth decay can begin.

Tooth decay is caused by a combination of factors, including bacteria in the mouth; frequent snacking; frequent sipping of sodas, fruit juice, and other sugary beverages; and inadequate brushing and other oral hygiene measures. *Cavities* are permanently damaged areas in the hard surface of the teeth that develop into tiny openings or holes. If left untreated, cavities get larger and affect deeper layers of the teeth. This can lead to severe toothache, infection, and ultimately, tooth loss. When cavities begin, there are usually no symptoms at all. But as the decay worsens, it can cause the following problems:

- Brown, black, or white staining on tooth surfaces.
- Pain that occurs in response to cold, hot, or sweet fluids and foods.
- Pain that occurs when you bite down.
- Toothache that is experienced all the time.
- Visible holes or pits in your teeth.

When tooth decay leads to tooth loss in children, it can contribute to the development of crooked teeth. Tooth loss can also lead to loss of social relationships, shame, embarrassment, and low self- esteem. This often is a cause of isolation, depression, and lack of social skills in adults and children. Tooth loss also leads to problems such as a reduced chewing capacity due to a lack of force and bite. When a patient loses a tooth, the opposing one can be displaced from its socket. This causes undesired contact with other teeth, leading to cavities, gum problems, and further damage. Often, the pain from such dental problems is debilitating. This is why it's so important to have good oral hygiene that discourages tooth decay and to schedule regular checkups so that cavities are identified and fixed at the earliest possible stage.

GUM DISEASE

Tooth decay and loss are the most obvious signs of poor oral health. But very often, there is another aspect of oral disease—gum disorders. This is a serious matter and a leading cause of tooth loss.

As mentioned earlier, plaque and tartar are ideally removed once or twice a year during conventional dental visits. This protects patients from many diseases and helps prevent the spread of bacteria within the mouth. Many people underestimate plaque and its lethal implications. *Plaque* is a sticky film that forms on teeth when bacteria in the mouth mix with sugary or starchy foods. It contains millions of bacteria. Plaque can be removed through brushing and flossing, but if it is not removed, it hardens into *tartar*. Also known as *calculus*, this substance forms above and below the gum line. Because tartar buildup is strongly bonded to the tooth enamel, it can be removed only by a dental professional. Unlike plaque, which is hard to see, tartar takes on a yellowish or brownish color. In many cases, you can feel and see tartar on the teeth. The longer plaque and tartar remain on your teeth, the more damage they can do. Both of these substances can cause gum disease. Below, we discuss first gingivitis, which is a relatively mild gum disease, and periodontitis, which is more advanced.

Gingivitis

If plaque isn't adequately removed, it builds up at the gum line and often results in *gingivitis,* or inflammation of the gums (or the gingiva). Gingivitis symptoms can include the following:

- Dark red gums.

- Gums that are irritated and bleed easily during brushing and flossing.

- Bad breath.

- Receding gums.

- Swollen or puffy gums

- Tender gums

Because of lack of knowledge about the importance of dental care, many Black Americans suffer from gingivitis well before earning their high school diploma and reaching adulthood. It is important to understand that plaque can be easily removed through self-care. However, if you are experiencing the symptoms of gingivitis, it's vital to immediately seek the help of a dentist before gingivitis progresses to periodontitis.

Periodontitis

As time progresses, untreated gingivitis advances into a gum disease known as periodontitis. A serious infection, *periodontitis* damages the gums and, without treatment, can harm the bone and connective tissue around the teeth. In severe cases, this can lead to the loosening of teeth and tooth loss.

While gingivitis is curable, typically, the effects of periodontitis are not reversible. It is a chronic, long-term condition that must be addressed with the help of a dental professional.

OTHER ORAL PROBLEMS

Oral problems other than tooth decay and gum disease can occur for a variety of reasons, including inadequate hygiene, lowered immunity, and irritation caused by habits such as smoking. The following are some of the problems that you may experience. If you see or feel something unusual on your gums or elsewhere in your mouth, it is important to bring it to the attention of your dentist or another healthcare provider so that the disorder can be immediately diagnosed and treated.

Leukoplakia

Leukoplakia is a condition that causes white patches or plaques to develop on your gums, the insides of your cheeks, the bottom of your mouth, and sometimes your tongue. These patches cannot be scraped off.

Doctors don't know exactly what causes leukoplakia, but they consider mouth irritants such as smoking to be the main culprit in its development. Most leukoplakia patches are noncancerous, but they may indicate a potential for cancer. If you develop patches such as this, it is best to see your dentist or physician to evaluate the problem.

Mouth Sores

Mouth sores can appear on any of the soft tissues of the mouth, including the gums, cheeks, floor and roof of the mouth, tongue, and lips. These sores can even develop on the esophagus, which is the tube that leads to your stomach.

Mouth sores are usually a minor irritation that last a week or two and then heal. Canker sores, which are quite common, fall into this category of annoying (and painful) but usually minor sores that do not require treatment. However, in some cases, sores can indicate a more serious infection or even mouth cancer. If an unusual sore appears on your mouth and fails to go way within a week or two, be sure to pay a visit to your dentist.

Oral Thrush

Also known as *candidiasis* or simply *thrush*, *oral thrush* occurs when a yeast infection develops inside the mouth, causing white or yellowing bumps to form on the inner cheeks and tongue. This most often occurs in infants and toddlers, and usually goes away on its own. However, oral thrush can also be experienced by adults, with symptoms including soreness or burning in the mouth; a

THE FAILURE OF THE MEDICAL COMMUNITY TO RAISE AWARENESS OF ORAL HEALTH

Medical doctors rarely advise patients of the need for better dental care—despite the fact that a doctor should be able to see that dental care is required simply by looking in the patient's mouth. Medical officials are failing to educate and inquire about the spread and results of gum disease. Even worse, the CDC released a study stating that more than 80 percent of internal medicine trainees never ask patients if they have been diagnosed with periodontitis. Perhaps this is not surprising, since 90 percent of these professionals did not receive any medical school training about periodontal disease and the systemic link to African Americans. Finally, more than 40 percent of these physicians believe that discussing periodontal disease is not related to their roles.

Clearly, doctors should be better trained to consider the health of the total person and to understand that oral health reflects the well-being of the body. (See the discussion on page 221 to learn about disorders that are associated with poor oral health.) In the meantime, it is vital for patients to take responsibility for their own oral hygiene and, when necessary, to seek the help of a dentist or other qualified professional.

cotton-like sensation in the mouth; dry, cracked skin at the corners of the mouth; a bad taste; or loss of taste.

The most common cause of oral thrush in adults is improper removal and cleaning of an upper denture. Other potential causes include taking antibiotics, having a compromised immune system, and diabetes. Fortunately, your doctor can treat this condition with a range of antifungal medications.

FOOD AND ORAL DISEASES

Food is at the heart of African-American culture. When we get together, we love to pull out the grill and the cooler. We fill our coolers with chilled Coke, Sprite, Pepsi, high-sugar juices, and other sweet beverages. Grandma whips up the potato salad, and we all have an uncle who loves to season up the beef and pork ribs before putting them on the grill. And, of course, a cookout wouldn't be complete with a sweet treat for dessert. Cooking and eating is how we express love.

The problem lies in the fact that a poor diet is one of the leading causes of oral disease. They are all related. As a community, we have to come together and decide what is most important—sticking to much-loved but unhealthy traditions, or making changes that will lead to a longer, healthier life. We can still gather together, but perhaps we should limit starches and sweets to one or two per meal. Try adding some vegetable salads with nonsweet dressings to the table. When it comes to both good oral health and blood sugar control, it's also vital to avoid sugary drinks. Just as important, after eating, be sure to brush your teeth and remove the sugar and starchy residues that promote plaque. (For more tips on good oral care, see the discussion on page 225.)

HEALTH DISORDERS ASSOCIATED WITH POOR ORAL HEALTH

The mouth is home to about 700 species of bacteria, including bacteria that can cause gum disease. Clearly, the mouth is connected to the rest of the body, and as oral bacteria breaks into the bloodstream, it can travel to organs throughout the body. This is why taking care of oral health benefits not just your gums and your teeth, but also your general health. Telltale symptoms of oral problems—such as puffy gums or blood in the sink after brushing—should lead you to take remedial measures that may actually help prevent a range of quite serious disorders. If you neglect your mouth, your body will suffer. And if your general health is suffering, it can have an adverse impact on your oral health, causing a vicious cycle. Following are some of the health problems that have been linked to poor oral health.

Alzheimer's Disease

Study results published in the *Journal of Alzheimer's Disease* suggest that the bacteria that cause gum disease are also associated with the development of Alzheimer's disease and related dementia, particularly vascular dementia. Bacteria and the inflammatory substances they make can travel from infections in the mouth through the bloodstream and finally to the brain. The study showed that older adults with signs of gum disease and oral infections are more likely to develop Alzheimer's disease than are older adults with better oral hygiene.

Cancer

Evidence suggests that chronic infection and inflammation in the mouth, as seen in people whose teeth and gums are in poor condition, is associated with an increased risk of cancer development. Some studies have indicated that poor oral hygiene, especially when paired with smoking, are associated with certain mouth and throat cancers. Poor oral health has also been linked with a greatly increased risk of hepatocellular carcinoma, the most common form of liver cancer.

Cardiovascular Disease

Study after study has shown that people with poor oral health—such as tooth loss or gum disease—have higher rates of heart attack and stroke than people with good oral health. This association may be due to at least two factors. First, the bacteria that infect the gums also travel through the blood vessels, where they can cause damage and inflammation within the vessels. Blood clots, heart attack, and stroke may follow. Second, the body's immune response to the oral inflammation may result in a cascade of vascular damage throughout the body.

Diabetes

Research has shown that gum disease may increase the risk of diabetes, because the presence of periodontal disease affects blood sugar control. Moreover, individuals with diabetes are twice as likely to develop periodontal disease as individuals without diabetes. In the United States, one out of every five cases of total tooth loss is associated with diabetes.

Eating Disorders

Often, dentists are the first professionals to notice an eating disorder, because this problem is often signaled by bad breath, inflamed gums, sensitive teeth, and tooth erosion. Without proper nutrition, gums and other soft tissues inside the mouth bleed easily. The glands that produce saliva can also swell, causing the individual to experience chronic dry mouth. Eventually, the jaw bone can weaken, which weakens the teeth and leads to tooth loss.

When patients have bulimia, harsh stomach acid from frequent vomiting erodes tooth enamel, increasing the risk of tooth decay. The color, shape, and length of the teeth may all be affected, and the edges of the teeth can become thin and break off easily.

High Blood Pressure

Research has shown that red, tender, or bleeding gums can trigger high blood pressure. When gums are infected, the disease can spread to other parts of the body, causing systemic inflammation that eventually damages blood vessels. In a review of numerous studies, scientists found that people who had moderate gum disease had a 22-percent increased risk for high blood pressure, and those with severe gum disease had a nearly 50-percent higher risk. In several studies, blood pressure dropped when the gum disease was treated.

Kidney Disease

Just as research has shown that inflammation due to periodontal disease can affect the heart, it has shown that inflammation in the mouth can put kidneys at risk. Moreover, over time, the gum bacteria causing an infection in the mouth can spread to other organs of the body, including the kidneys, resulting in life-threatening infections. Although more study is needed, the possibility of kidney disease is an excellent reason to maintain healthy gums and teeth.

Pneumonia and Other Respiratory Infections

There is a clear connection between poor oral health and respiratory disease. When bacteria grow out of control in the mouth, and gingivitis or other oral infections go untreated, the bacteria can be breathed into the lungs or can travel there via the bloodstream. Once there, the bacteria can lead to pneumonia and bronchitis and can worsen conditions such as emphysema. Although a healthy immune system can fight off unhealthy bacteria, an immune system that is already taxed because of oral health issues is more likely to allow tissues in other portions of the body to become irritated, inflamed, and infected.

Rheumatoid Arthritis

Since the early 1900s, medical investigators have observed an association between gum disease and rheumatoid arthritis (RA), and over time, researchers have suspected that both diseases may be triggered by a common factor. The bacteria *Porphyromonas gingivalis* is known to be involved in the serious gum disease periodontitis. Because this same bacteria has been found to trigger or worsen RA, it has been suggested that when the bacteria are allowed to grow unchecked in the mouth, they cause certain immune system proteins to become overactive, which eventually harms the joints. RA patients are significantly more likely to have gum disease, and it has been found that when gum disease is severe, RA disease has increased activity.

If you were not already aware of how a lack of dental care can lead to serious medical conditions, you are not alone. Too many people, Black and White, don't realize that neglect of oral health can have serious consequences. Fortunately, there is much you can do to increase the well-being of your teeth and gums. The following section looks at the easy steps you can take.

TIPS FOR BETTER ORAL CARE

To avoid dental disease and the many serious disorders that can follow, it is important to establish good preventive dental care. Preventive care is so much more than regular checkups. It starts in early childhood, when dental professionals can teach you and your child how to brush correctly. The dentist or assistant can also discuss what foods and beverages build strong teeth and what foods and beverages will cause cavities and dental disease.

Preventive care is built on habits. As parents and caregivers, it is our duty to correct the misinformation and bad habits that may have been passed on to us. Adopting and teaching habits like brushing your teeth every day and night with non-abrasive toothpastes is a prime example of how habits that can make or break your oral health. Below are a number of good habits you can adopt and teach—involving regular checkups, a good oral hygiene regimen, diet, and more—that will help prevent both oral problems and more serious health disorders.

Get Regular Dental Care

- **TAKE YOUR CHILDREN TO THE DENTIST WHEN THEY GET THEIR FIRST TEETH.** Make the first visit fun so your kids can become familiar with the dentist. Remember—and tell your children—that the first visit is simply a healthy dental visit.

- **VISIT THE DENTIST TWICE A YEAR.** Your own everyday habits are crucial to your overall oral health. Still, even the most dutiful brushers and flossers need to see a dentist regularly. At minimum, you should see your dentist for cleanings and checkups twice a year.

- **ASK YOUR DENTIST AND/OR HIS ASSISTANT TO HELP YOU FORM GOOD DENTAL HABITS.** During checkups, ask for advice regarding the best toothpaste, toothbrush, and brushing and flossing techniques for you. Also ask about other devices, such as special picks, that can help improve your oral health.

Establish Good Oral Hygiene Habits

- **DON'T GO TO BED WITHOUT BRUSHING YOUR TEETH.** Everything you have eaten is still on your teeth at night before you go to bed, and sleep provides the perfect warm, moist, dark environment to promote the growth of bacteria. By brushing before you go to bed, you will prevent your mouth from becoming a breeding ground for bacterial growth.

- **USE A TOOTHPASTE THAT CONTAINS FLUORIDE.** Fluoride comes from an element in the earth's soil called fluorine. Many experts believe that fluoride helps prevent cavities, and it is a common ingredient in toothpaste and mouthwash. However, some dental products do not contain fluoride. Evidence suggests that a lack of fluoride can lead to tooth decay even if the individual brushes properly.

- **CHANGE YOUR TOOTHBRUSH OFTEN.** Bristles deteriorate with time and usage, so if you're using the same toothbrush beyond a few months, you may not be getting the best clean anymore. Dentists will often offer free toothbrushes to their patients. Replace your brush when your dentist gives you a new one or whenever you see the bristles splaying out.

- **DON'T NEGLECT YOUR TONGUE.** Your tongue holds onto plaque and bacteria like a sponge. Always use a tongue scraper for your tongue or brush it with your toothbrush. If you neglect this aspect of oral care, the bacterial growth can cause gum disease, tooth decay, and bad breath.

- **REMEMBER THAT FLOSSING IS JUST IMPORTANT AS BRUSHING.** If you do not floss your teeth, you are only removing half of plaque and bacteria, because half of it is stuck between your teeth. If allowed to remain there, it will affect your gums and your breath. If you or your children find flossing difficult, try plastic picks and other flossing aids.

- **USE MOUTHWASH.** Mouthwash helps in many ways. It reduces the amount of acid in the mouth; it helps clean hard-to-reach areas in and around the gums; and, if you use a mouthwash that contains fluoride, it remineralizes the teeth. Mouthwash can also be helpful against bad breath or dry mouth, depending on the brand you choose.

Make Dietary Changes That Promote Oral Health

- **LIMIT SUGARY AND ACIDIC FOODS.** Ultimately, sugar converts into acid in the mouth, which can then erode the enamel of your teeth. These acids are what lead to cavities. Acidic fruits, teas, and coffee can also wear down tooth enamel. While you don't necessarily have to avoid such foods altogether, it doesn't hurt to be mindful and limit their consumption.

- **EAT CRUNCHY FRUITS AND VEGETABLES.** Crisp fruits and raw vegetables—apples, carrots, and celery, for instance—help clean plaque from teeth and freshen your breath. Many fruits and vegetables also contain antioxidant compounds, such as vitamin C, that help protect the gums and other oral tissues from cellular damage and bacterial infection.

- **DRINK WATER.** Drinking water after you eat helps wash away some of the sticky and acidic foods that cling to your teeth after you eat, causing decay and eroding enamel. Water is also good for overall health.

Eliminate Habits That Can Harm Teeth and Gums

- **DO NOT SMOKE.** Smoking harms the body's immune system, which makes it difficult for the body to heal tissues, including those in the mouth. The CDC names smoking as a risk factor for gum disease, while the American Dental Association warns that people who smoke may experience slow healing after a dental procedure. Smoking is an irritant that can cause mouth sores or other problems. Smoking also affects the appearance of the mouth, leading to yellowing of the teeth and tongue, and can cause bad breath.

- **DO NOT BITE YOUR NAILS.** Biting your fingernails causes serious damage not only to the hands, but also to your teeth. Teeth are not meant to withstand the damage of nail biting, and most individuals have no idea just how many bacteria they are introducing to their mouths when they bite their nails.

- **DO NOT CHEW ICE.** One of the most damaging things you can do to your teeth is to chew ice. Using your teeth to break ice down can cause the surface of the tooth to crack and break, wearing down the enamel and making the tooth more susceptible to further damage, like cavities. Eating ice can also ruin fillings, as ice causes the filling to expand, shortening its life span and increasing sensitivity. Other risks associated with chewing ice include damaged gums, headaches, toothaches, and soreness in the jaw.

- **STOP GRINDING YOUR TEETH AND CLENCHING YOUR JAW.** Grinding teeth and clenching the jaw are detrimental to your oral health. Many people do not even realize that they are participating in these habits, especially if they do so only in their sleep. Grinding teeth is most commonly a result of stress, anxiety, or an improper bite alignment. When sleep grinding occurs, the jaw exerts three to ten times more force than when chewing and breaking down food. This can cause tooth mobility, cracking, or breaking. The teeth can also be ground down, causing sensitivity.

Make Sure You Get Adequate Vitamin D

- **GET SOME SUN AND TAKE VITAMIN D SUPPLEMENTS.** Vitamin D plays a crucial role in the regulation of both calcium and phosphorus levels in the bloodstream, which are two important factors in the development and maintenance of strong, healthy bones and teeth. If you lack vitamin D, you are at risk of developing a calcium deficiency, which can contribute to underdeveloped teeth, tooth decay, and gum diseases like gingivitis. In more severe cases, calcium deficiency can result in periodontal disease, which affects not only the gums but also the periodontal ligaments and alveolar bones of the teeth, which directly support the teeth. While spending time in the sun can help ensure your body's production of D3, most people need to get D from supplements. Take 2,000 IU to 5,000 IU per day of vitamin D3. You can also ask your healthcare provider to test your vitamin D levels and prescribe a dosage based on your test results. Make sure that your physician orders the 25-OH vitamin D test, as this will give you the best indication of your vitamin D body stores.

Remember that black mouths matter. While you are establishing better habits, talk to your family and friends about the importance of oral health.

ORAL DISPARITIES IN THE AFRICAN-AMERICAN COMMUNITY

Oral health is often poor in African-American communities and is linked to many common diseases, such as heart disease, stroke, and diabetes. Adults of minority descent are at a high risk of having poor oral health due to inadequate access to health services, particularly dental care. Children suffer, too. Two systemic issues contribute to oral neglect in Black communities—poverty and discrimination. African Americans in the United States are more likely to be uninsured due to low income. Without insurance, Black Americans face considerable barriers to receiving health services. The following discussions will look at the effects of poverty and racism on dental care in the Black community and will examine the problems of black children in particular. Finally, we discuss what you can do to get affordable dental care.

Poverty and Insurance

It's important to point out that almost half of the African-American community is using Medicaid for insurance. Government-funded dental preventive and treatment services are sparse if you are on Medicaid, with individual states determining what dental care, if any, is available in their state. That explains why coverage varies so greatly across the United States. Add to that the fact that those on Medicaid cannot afford health insurance, let alone the additional copayment fees that accompany procedures not covered by Medicaid. The fact is that if you are on Medicaid, your coverage is very limited.

Studies have shown that health insurance coverage varies substantially between racial and ethnic groups in the United States. Compared with Whites, African Americans have persistently lower insurance coverage for certain standard procedures at all ages. Racial and ethnic disparities in health insurance coverage rates account for a sizable share of healthcare access difference.

Many healthcare providers require insurance coverage from their patients or charge unaffordable fees that are to be paid before service is rendered. Patients are screened for insurance stability. Imagine being discriminated against because you could not afford insurance in the past despite presently having insurance. Inconsistent or unstable insurance coverage has negative consequences. Patients who frequently change healthcare providers due to insurance discrepancies or payment delays experience more interruptions in their care. They are also less likely to establish ongoing relationships with their physicians.

Racial Barriers

Racial barriers and discrimination within the healthcare community discourage low-income African Americans from using a wide range of needed health services, including dental services. Similarly, individuals who have experienced racism are 25 percent less likely to visit the dentist than those who have not. In a study that focused on caregivers' experiences in accessing dental care for their children, African-American participants explicitly pointed to racial discrimination as a "major barrier" in seeking care.

The Children of Low-Income Families

Adults are not the only group who suffer from poverty. Children of low-income families also bear the injustice of America's social system. Low-income Black children of ages two to eleven experience 60 percent untreated cavities in comparison to high-income families at 46 percent. As an ineffective way to cope with unmet needs, Black households commonly ignore telltale signs of failing oral health. If your eye started bleeding after you rubbed it, wouldn't you find it necessary to go to the doctor? Why isn't the same reaction common when someone notices that their gums are bleeding after brushing their teeth? We have grown numb to irregular behaviors as a way to cope with poverty and disparity. The results of this disparity, generally, become evident in childhood, with African-American children's rate of untreated dental cavities almost triple that of their White peers by the time they reach their teens.

Hispanic children experience tooth decay at even higher rates than White and African-American children. Think about this: Studies have shown that the first dental visit for a White child is between three and five years of age. The average age for the first dental visit for African-American children is twelve, and for Hispanic children, sixteen.

What makes this so heartbreaking is that the twelve-year-old African-American child and sixteen-year-old Hispanic child are probably at the dentist because of tooth pain. Addressing tooth-ache pain is distressing for most children. They face condemnation for the state of their oral health. As you could imagine, this is not a good experience for any child, especially for the first visit. It is mentally scarring and sets the tone for future visits.

Of course, a better strategy is to start medical checkups at an earlier age and either prevent tooth decay or catch it at an early stage, before it becomes painful. Below, we look at ways in which you can gain access to dental care that you can afford.

How to Obtain Access to Dental Care

Not only your oral health but also your general health depend on your finding affordable, quality dental care for yourself and your family. But as you know, dental procedures—even the examination and set of x-rays used to diagnose a problem—can be pricey. Here are some suggestions for finding a good affordable dentist:

- Talk to the people you know about dentists in the area. Start by asking your friends if they have had a positive dental experience and could recommend a dentist. Also ask around at work. Tell your primary care physician, or perhaps the nurse at the doctor's office, that you are interested in taking better care of your mouth, and ask for a reference. Also enquire if your pastor knows of a skilled dentist who is taking patients.

- Call your Community Health Department and ask if they have a list of dentists they can recommend. You may have a government dental clinic located near you. Most states offer free or low-cost facilities that provide dental care.

- If your city has a dental school attached to a university, call and ask if they are accepting patients. Dental students need practice before they can acquire a dental license, but the students are supervised by a fully qualified dentist.

- If you are homebound or a senior citizen, you may be eligible for care at a Mobile Dental Clinic. This means that the dental office will come to you! The staff of a Mobile Dental Clinic can clean your teeth, repair any cavities, pull any teeth that are beyond saving, and tell you how to care for your teeth. Here, too, you can check with your Community Health Department to see if such a service is available.

- Some communities or charitable organizations provide low-cost or free dental clinics. Local dentists volunteer their time and provide good-quality dental care free of charge or at an affordable price. Ask your pastor, your doctor, and your Community Health Department if such opportunities are available near you.

- If you are on Medicaid, perform an online search for "dentist who accepts Medicaid patients" in your town or city. You can also contact your Community Health Department to see if they can provide you with some local dentists who accept Medicaid.

- If you are suffering from severe pain or suspect you have a serious dental infection, you can always go to your hospital emergency room. They may have a dentist on call who will extract the tooth for free and, if needed, provide antibiotics. Before you leave this dentist, ask if he or she can recommend a dentist who would accept you at a price you can afford. While Medicare does not cover most dental care, dental procedures, or supplies, like cleanings, fillings, tooth extractions, dentures, dental plates, or other dental devices, under Medicare Part A (Hospital Insurance), it will pay for certain dental services that are available when you are in a hospital. Part A can pay for inpatient hospital care if you need to have emergency or complicated dental procedures, even though the dental care isn't covered.

CONCLUSION

Now you know about the dental issues our community faces every day, and why it's so important to take care of your mouth—not only so that you will have strong teeth and healthy gums, but because good oral health promotes good overall health. To follow the recommendations in this chapter, you need to find a regular dentist that you and your family like. This professional can help you and your children care for your mouth and teeth. See your dentist every six months, and be sure to brush and floss daily. Take charge of your oral health just as you manage other aspects of your well-being. Like Maya Angelou said, "Do the best you can until you know better. Then when you know better, do better." Let's all do better!

TIMELINES
THE IMMORTAL CANCER CELL

One of the major breakthroughs in cancer research was the discovery of a human cancer cell that was immortal. In 1951, biologist George Gey working at Johns Hopkins Hospital discovered a cervical cancer cell that could be kept alive for as long as needed. Before the discovery, researchers could work only on cervical cancer cells that had been recently extracted from cancer patients. This cell was named the HeLa cancer cell. With the discovery of this one type of immortal cell, researchers began to look for other HeLa cells in various other types of cancers, and as time went on, they found them. These were called cell lines and could now be used in ongoing cancer research.

The HeLa cell was named after the woman who was the source of the cell, Henrietta Lacks, a thirty-one-year-old African-American woman from Maryland. After suffering severe abdominal pain, she was admitted to Johns Hopkins Hospital, the only hospital in her area that would treat Black patients. It was discovered she had cervical cancer. During her treatments, two samples of her cervical cells were taken without her knowledge. Three months later, she passed away. It was these samples that allowed George Gey to make his discovery. However, the source of these cells was not fully revealed to the family for thirty years. Today, we recognize that it was Henrietta Lacks, a woman of color, who helped cancer research take an important step forward.

Conclusion

"Of all the forms of inequality, injustice in health is the most shocking and inhuman."
—Dr. Martin Luther King, Jr.

In every chapter of this book, I have attempted to weave together aspects of diseases that have historically plagued us, and connect these with the issues of life we face every day as African Americans. For every disease condition, there are causes that cross over many lines. These include our history, culture and traditions, diets, environment, and beliefs, and it's these areas of our lives that allow for these conditions to occur. Few if any of the diseases covered in this book stand alone. The occurrence of cancer has specific causes that predict and support its existence. The same is true for cardiovascular disease, diabetes, hypertension, kidney disease, and the rest. They are interdependent.

Looking at any disease condition without exploring associated facts strips people's ability to help solve their own healthcare issues. In traditional medicine, every condition is thought to be a separate, isolated disease, without the interactions of the body's conditions and surrounding environments. What I hope you have come to understand is the underlying principle on which I've based my own practice—functional medicine. In *functional medicine*, patients and practitioners work together to address the underlying causes of disease and promote optimal wellness. In other words, the whole person and his or her entire life must always be considered in the prevention and treatment of health conditions.

Empowerment is the goal of this book. We should no longer need to be afraid of any disease, believing that there's nothing we can do to prevent it or eliminate it. Nor should we be completely dependent on providers, clinics, and various healthcare institutions to determine the fate of our health. The state of our health should be a shared responsibility, and the care of our health involves a partnership. As a patient or caretaker, you need to understand the problem, ask the right questions, and, just as important, make informed decisions. Does this mean that if you did everything correctly, you would never become sick? No, it does not. What it does mean is that we all, to a great degree, have it within ourselves to control the state of our health.

As a community, we must learn from the past. We must pay closer attention to our own health and that of our family. We must never accept a healthcare system that has shown itself to underservice our communities. That's how we got here—with an American healthcare model built on the backs of our people. It stole our bodies in death, it kidnapped us, it performed surgical procedures without available anesthesia, and it experimented on us without scientific purpose. We must never let this happen again

However, with that said, it does not mean you should not use the healthcare system that exists. It does not mean avoiding your annual exam. On the contrary, you should do whatever you must to obtain the preventive care required to maintain your health. Not doing anything to help yourself means you're allowing disease to take hold rather than preventing it.

THE AMERICAN HEALTHCARE SYSTEM

We are all used to hearing about the United States healthcare "system"—how it works for some, but not for others. The truth is that the healthcare system we have is not a unified system. The vast majority of our hospitals, clinics, and doctors' practices belong to for-profit healthcare companies that work independently of one another. Compare that to banking in the United States. You can go to any ATM in any city in this country—or the world—and get money from your bank or credit card. That's a system. Try getting your medical records or your lab results to another doctor when you need them. It won't happen. This is just one cause of the dysfunctionality of our "system" and of why healthcare is offered unequally to different communities based on race and social status.

Over the last twenty years, American medicine has made huge technical strides in nearly every component of healthcare—in electronic medical records, telemedicine, remote surgical procedures, and the list goes on. However, it has never examined the poorer care given to African Americans, nor has it made concrete plans about what can and should be changed going forward. As more history has come to light, it has become known that many of medicine's advancements have been made by doctors, students, and researchers through the cruel treatment of Black men and women. Today, people of color receive less care—and worse care—than White Americans.

Unfortunately, none of this is taught in today's medical schools. It has never been part of the curriculum offered to students, interns, residents, or fellows in training. Therefore, each successive class comes and goes the same way they have since the Royal Hospital, the first true hospital, was established in New Orleans, Louisiana in 1722. Most doctors are oblivious to the historical treatment of African Americans. If they enter medical school with any ingrained prejudices, these attitudes are likely to remain in place. Unfortunately, these attitudes significantly affect the way patients are diagnosed and treated.

RACIAL DISPARITY

Although the problem of racial disparity in healthcare is well known, there is no clear plan or commitment to address it, let alone fix it. Specifically, we are talking about *implicit bias*—unconscious attitudes and stereotypes towards groups. At its worse, implicit bias in healthcare costs lives and increases suffering. With the stakes so high, if implicit bias should be confronted in any area of American life, it should certainly be confronted in healthcare.

Although most healthcare professionals know that there is no equity in healthcare, rather than saying anything, they simply accept the status quo. This attitude reinforces the institutional racism experienced by Black Americans every day. However, it's important to understand that what we see in healthcare reflects the prevailing attitude in our society in general.

In 1865, a civil war fought to free the slaves ended, and while the Emancipation Proclamation pronounced African Americans "free," to a great degree, we were still second-class citizens. It was the Black civil rights movement of the 1960s lead by Martin Luther King, Jr. and others that began to shatter the Jim Crow laws intended to "keep us in our place." Yet sixty years later, we continue to experience racial discrimination and inequality. My hope is that there will be change for the better. The question is: How fast will it come?

Unfortunately, the attitudes of today's healthcare professionals, on any level, are unlikely to be changed until major changes are made in society for Black Americans. This is a nice way of saying, "Don't hold your breath."

In a 2000 study on racial disparities published in the *Medicare & Medicaid Research Review*, Drs. David R. Williams and Toni D. Rucker concluded the following:

> It is a national embarrassment that there are large and persisting racial differences in health. National data reveal, for example, that black persons had an overall mortality rate that was 1.6 times higher than white persons in 1995—identical to the black/white mortality ratio in 1950. Moreover, for multiple causes of death (heart disease, cancer, diabetes, and cirrhosis of the liver) the racial discrepancy was larger in 1995 than in 1950. These inequities fly in the face of cherished American principles given the public's commitment to principles of equal treatment in society. As a society, we need to make it a national priority to build on the cultural support for egalitarian principles and develop strategies to eradicate racial inequities in medical care.

This leads us to an important question: What can we, as people of color, do to improve the health of our family and community? The answer lies in the realization that we have the power to control our own lives.

EMPOWERMENT

This is a pivotal time for African Americans—a time that has given birth to a national movement called Black Lives Matter. The movement rose in response to the May 2020 video of a police officer's knee on the neck of George Floyd, and led to marches and protests in cities throughout this country. Not since the 1960s have we seen such a dramatic response to an act of cruelty. Unfortunately, Floyd's death is only one of many Black deaths that have occurred at the hands of police. These unnecessary killings have long been commonplace in our communities, forcing mothers and fathers to give their children "the talk," which explains how the child should act when confronted by law enforcement. But until the Floyd video, most White people seemed oblivious to the problem. Now this issue, as well as other related racially-based problems, is making national headlines.

While it is important to point out that these marches were composed of both Blacks and Whites, something else seemed to be occurring in our communities. Blacks began to register to vote in record numbers—first in the thousands, and then in the millions. By going out and voting as a block, we prevented the election of politicians who believed that Black lives are of no value. This ability to determine who will be running our local, state, and national governments is vital for our future. It enables us to make our voices heard and to make change.

If our various systems of healthcare are failing us, we now have an opportunity to have our politicians represent our interests. It may have taken us over one hundred and fifty years to get here, but we are here. There is no doubt that racism will not disappear, but understanding and using the power we have in our hands can overcome many of these obstacles. If we can make it clear that healthcare is a right and not a privilege—for Black people as well as White, for the poor as well as the rich—we will have taken a giant step in the right direction.

RESPONSIBILITY

It's vital to create greater equality in our nation's healthcare system. But it's also vital for us to take responsibility for our own health and for the behavior that helps shape our well-being. Too many of us seem to be surprised when a doctor explains that the symptoms we are experiencing are caused by an underlying condition that could end our lives. If you have read all of the previous chapters in this book, it should definitely not come as a surprise. The stats don't lie. Each year, millions of us are dying before our time, and that should not be happening. Too many of us ignore the symptoms until it's too late to effectively treat the problem. As you have learned, there are many simple things you can do to avoid some of the most common disorders that confront us. And it's not that hard.

You need to take responsibility for your own health. While you may not be able to avoid racist behavior on the part of others, you need to know if incidents with racist people raise your blood pressure to a dangerous level. Or is it the fast food that's causing that problem—or the lack of exercise? Or worse, could it be that all of these factors have made you vulnerable to the silent killer of hypertension?

By taking steps to avoid developing high blood pressure or to lower it if you already have it, you take on a responsibility that can add years to your life. And when you go to a doctor, you need to share the responsibility for your health. If you don't understand something your doctor says, ask questions. If you learn that you have a health disorder, read up on it. See what you can do on your own to improve your condition. Even as a patient, you have more power than you think. Use it.

CONCLUSION

For too long, racism has played too great a role in our community and our lives. It is not going away tomorrow, but things are changing. Do you remember when practically every TV commercial featured a White man or woman? It wasn't that long ago when ads were aimed at the audience that White advertising agents believed were mostly likely to consume their clients' products. It was also a subtle way of saying that only the White audience mattered. Too often, Black woman were given the impression that to be beautiful, they needed to have straight hair and light complexions. Whether or not this was done on purpose, the use of only White actors on commercials marginalized us.

Today, things have changed considerably. Commercials now feature Black couples, mixed-race couples, Hispanic couples, Asian couples, and gay couples. For the first time, ads reflect who we are as a nation. This is important, because these are the people your children will see on TV—and this will likely transform attitudes. But this is still only one element of our society. We have to make many changes in many areas. Whatever lies ahead, change must begin with who we are and what we choose to do on a personal level to improve our lives.

Glossary

Occasionally, this book may use terms that are not familiar to you. You may also hear these terms when working with doctors and other healthcare professionals. To help you better understand and participate in discussions with your physician, definitions are provided below for words that are often used by those in the fields of health and nutrition. All terms that appear in *italic type* are also defined within the glossary.

ACANTHOSIS NIGRICANS. A skin condition characterized by darkened areas of skin around the neck or armpits. The affected skin can become thickened.

ACE INHIBITORS (ANGIOTENSIN CONVERTING ENZYME INHIBITORS). Medications that inhibit (slow) the activity of the blood vessel-narrowing enzyme ACE, thereby causing blood vessels to enlarge or dilate so that *blood pressure* is reduced.

ADIPOCYTOKINES. A family of cell-signaling *hormones*, including *leptin* and *adiponectin,* that are secreted by fat (adipose) tissue. Adipocytokines affect glucose and fat metabolism, reproduction, and cardiovascular function.

ADIPONECTIN. A *hormone* secreted exclusively by fat (adipose) tissue that regulates the metabolism of lipids and glucose, increasing *insulin* sensitivity so that the body responds properly to blood sugar levels.

ADVANCED GLYCATION END PRODUCTS (AGES). Harmful compounds that are formed when protein or fat combines with sugar in the bloodstream. The production of AGEs is accelerated by the excess *blood glucose* characteristic of *diabetes.*

AEROBIC ACTIVITY. Brisk exercise that promotes the circulation of oxygen through the bloodstream and increases breathing and heart rates. Brisk walking, running, bicycling, and swimming are all aerobic activities.

AMINO ACIDS. The structural units, or building blocks, that the body uses to make the special proteins used to repair cells, to make new cells, and to grow and develop normally.

ANALGESIC NEPHROPATHY. Damage to one or both kidneys resulting from the long-term use of one or more pain medications (analgesics).

ANEMIA. A condition marked by a deficiency of healthy *red blood cells* or *hemoglobin,* the protein that carries oxygen in the blood.

ANTIBIOTICS. Medications, such as penicillin, that are designed to kill or inhibit the growth of harmful *bacteria* that enter the body and cause infection.

ANTIOXIDANTS. Substances, either natural or artificial, that can prevent or slow damage to cells caused by *free radicals,* unstable molecules that the body produces both during normal metabolic processes and as a reaction to environmental and other pressures.

ARB BLOCKERS (ANGIOTENSIN RECEPTOR BLOCKER). Medications that block the blood vessel-narrowing effects of the chemical angiotensin II, causing the blood vessels to enlarge or dilate so that *blood pressure* is reduced.

ARTERIES. Blood vessels that deliver oxygen-rich blood from the heart and lungs to the tissues of the body.

ASBESTOS. A fibrous material composed of six naturally occurring silicate minerals. Asbestos has been found to be carcinogenic and can lead to mesothelioma, a cancer of the thin membranes that line the chest and abdomen.

ATHEROSCLEROSIS. Narrowing and thickening of the *arteries* due to a buildup of *plaque*—deposits made up of fat, *cholesterol,* cellular waste products, calcium, and fibrin (a clotting material). The narrowed, hardened blood vessels reduce blood flow, lessening the amount of oxygen and other nutrients that reach the cells of the body. Atherosclerosis is also called hardening of the arteries.

ATRIAL FIBRILLATION. An irregular heartbeat of the heart's upper chambers (the atria) that can lead to blood clots, *stroke*, and other heart-related conditions.

BACTERIA. Microscopic organisms, not visible to the naked eye, that are found both inside and outside the body. Some bacteria are beneficial, and some can cause disease.

BETA CELLS. The cells in the pancreas that produce the hormone *insulin*.

BETA-BLOCKERS. Medications used to block the effect of the stress hormones norepinephrine and epinephrine (adrenaline), and thereby reduce heart rate and *blood pressure.*

BLOOD GLUCOSE. Also called blood sugar, the main sugar found in your blood. The blood carries glucose to all of the body's cells, where the glucose is converted into energy for use.

BLOOD PRESSURE. The pressure of circulating blood against the walls of the blood vessels. See also *diastolic pressure; hypertension; systolic pressure.*

BODY MASS INDEX (BMI). A measure of body fat based on height and weight that applies to adult men and women. The BMI calculation divides an adult's weight in kilograms by his or height in meters squared. A BMI between 25 and 29.9 indicates that the person is overweight, and a BMI between 30 and 39.9 indicates *obesity.*

BONE MARROW TRANSPLANT. A procedure that infuses healthy blood-forming *stem cells* into the body to replace damaged or diseased bone marrow.

BORDERLINE DIABETES. See *prediabetes.*

CALCIUM CHANNEL BLOCKERS. Medications that disrupt the movement of blood vessel-constricting calcium in the heart and *arteries,* thereby enlarging or dilating the arteries so that *blood pressure* is reduced.

CANCER. One of more than one hundred disorders in which abnormal cells divide without control and can invade nearby tissues. These abnormal cells can spread (metastasize) to other parts of the body through the blood, lymphatic system, and direct contact.

CANDIDIASIS. See *oral thrush.*

CAPILLARIES. Tiny blood vessels that connect the *arteries* to the *veins* and facilitate the exchange of materials, such as oxygen and nutrients, between the blood and tissue cells.

CARCINOGEN. A substance or agent—such as tobacco smoke or *asbestos*—that can cause *cancer* in humans by interacting with a cell's DNA and inducing genetic mutations.

CARDIOVASCULAR DISEASE (CVD). A general term for disorders of the heart and the blood vessels, including *atherosclerosis* (hardening of the arteries), irregularity of the heart rhythm, weakening of the heart, bulging or ballooning of the blood vessels, and many more conditions.

CELLULAR RECEPTORS. Protein molecules—found within the cells and embedded in the surface of the cell's membranes—that allow the cells to receive signals from other cells and from hormones.

CERVICAL DYSPLASIA. A condition in which abnormal cells are found in the cervix (the lower end of the uterus). This is most often caused by human papillomavirus (HPV).

CHOLESTEROL. A waxy lipid (fat) that is produced by the body and consumed in some foods, and circulates in the blood. Although some cholesterol is needed by the body, too much can collect on the walls of the blood vessels as *plaque* and lead to problems such as *heart attack* and *stroke*. There are two types of cholesterol: low-density lipoprotein (LDL) cholesterol, which takes cholesterol to the arteries; and high-density lipoprotein (HDL) cholesterol, which removes excess cholesterol from the body.

CHRONIC KIDNEY DISEASE (CKD). A disorder characterized by a gradual decrease in kidney function, which in turn can cause a host of health problems, including the accumulation of waste products, high blood pressure (*hypertension*), acidosis, and *anemia*. There are five stages of kidney disease, each of which is based on the individual's *glomerular filtration rate (GFR)*, which measures how well the kidneys are filtering the blood.

COLONOSCOPY. A procedure in which a flexible fiber-optic instrument is inserted in the rectum and snaked through the large intestine (colon) in order to detect changes or abnormalities in the colon.

COMPLETE BLOOD COUNT (CBC). A laboratory test that provides information about the cells in a person's blood, including counts of *white blood cells, red blood cells,* and platelets; the concentration of *hemoglobin;* and the *hematocrit* (the ratio of the volume of red blood cells to the total volume of the liquid part of the blood, or plasma).

COMPLETE PROTEIN. A food that contains all nine of the essential *amino acids* that your body must get from your diet.

COMPLEX CARBOHYDRATES. Carbohydrates composed of sugar molecules that are strung together in long, complex chains. Both simple and complex carbs are turned into *glucose* (blood sugar) in the body, where they are used as energy. But complex carbs digest more slowly, which helps control blood sugar levels. Complex carbs are also typically more nutritious and filling than simple carbs.

CORTISOL. The most important *hormone* that helps the body respond to *stress.*

DENTAL PLAQUE. See *plaque.*

DIABETES. A disorder in which the body's ability to produce or respond to the *hormone insulin* is impaired, resulting in an abnormal metabolism of carbohydrates and elevated levels of *glucose* (sugar) in the blood. See also *gestational diabetes; prediabetes; type 1 diabetes; type 2 diabetes.*

DIABETIC NEUROPATHY. A complication of *diabetes* in which high levels of blood glucose cause nerve damage. This condition can result in tingling, numbness, burning, or pain in the hands and feet.

DIABETIC RETINOPATHY. A complication of *diabetes* caused by damage to the blood vessels at the back of the eye. This condition can cause blurred vision, distorted vision, and sometimes blindness.

DIASTOLIC PRESSURE. The force exerted by blood on the *artery* walls while the heart is momentarily at rest between heartbeats.

DIETARY FIBER. Also called roughage, the part of plant foods that your body can't digest or absorb, but that nevertheless provides a host of benefits. The consumption of fiber helps nourish the growth of good bacteria, helps prevent surges in blood sugar levels, and improves digestion.

DIGITAL RECTAL EXAM (DRE). An examination of a man's lower rectum, pelvis, and lower belly for the purpose of detecting an enlarged prostate.

DIURETICS. Also called water pills, medications designed to increase the amount of water and salt eliminated from the body in the form of urine.

ENDOCRINE GLANDS. A system of glands that include the hypothalamus, pituitary, pineal, thyroid, parathyroid, thymus, adrenals, pancreas, ovaries (in women), and testes (in men). These glands secrete *hormones*, the body's chemical messengers that affect the function of every organ in the body.

END-STAGE RENAL DISEASE (ESRD). The last stage of chronic kidney disease, when the kidneys fail and the individual must get dialysis or a kidney transplant to survive.

ENVIRONMENTAL HEALTH. The branch of healthcare that focuses on the relationship between people and their environment.

FASTING BLOOD GLUCOSE TEST. A test that measures the level of *glucose* in the blood during a fast of eight to twelve hours.

FIBER. See *dietary fiber.*

FLAVONOIDS. Chemical compounds found naturally in fruits and vegetables, nuts, and herbs and spices, as well as in wine, tea, and dark chocolate. Powerful *antioxidants*, flavonoids help your body fight off harmful *free radicals*; reduce inflammatory reactions triggered by allergens, toxins, and other irritants; lower *blood pressure*; and generally help the body function more efficiently.

FOOD DESERT. An area that has limited access to affordable and nutritious food, including fresh fruit and vegetables. Instead, the shops in the area offer mostly dried, canned, and processed foods.

FOOD OASIS. An area that has high access to supermarkets and smaller shops which offer nutritious food, including fresh fruits and vegetables.

FREE RADICALS. Unstable molecules that can damage cells and promote aging and aging-related health problems, such as inflammation, heart disease, and *cancer.*

FUNCTIONAL MEDICINE. An individualized, patient-centered, science-based approach that focuses on identifying and addressing the root causes of a disease. In functional medicine, patients and practitioners work together to promote optimal wellness.

GASTROINTENTINAL TRACT. See *gut*.

GENE THERAPY. An experimental technique that uses genes to treat or prevent disease. It can involve replacing or inactivating a disease-causing gene or introducing a new or modified gene that can fight the disease.

GESTATIONAL DIABETES. A condition in which blood sugar levels become high during pregnancy.

GHRELIN. A *hormone* produced predominantly by the stomach that stimulates the appetite.

GI TRACT. See *gut*.

GINGIVITIS. A common, relatively mild form of gum disease that causes redness, irritation, and inflammation (swelling) of the gums (gingiva) around the base of the teeth.

GLOMERULAR FILTRATION RATE (GFR). A test designed to measure the level of kidney function.

GLOMERULUS. A tiny structure in a kidney's *nephron* that filters the blood through a network of small blood vessels (*capillaries*).

GLUCOSE. The simple sugar that circulates in your bloodstream and that your body can convert into energy.

GUT. Also called the gastrointestinal tract and GI tract, it begins at the mouth and includes all of the organs involved in the digestion and absorption of food—the mouth, esophagus, stomach, small and large intestines, anus, liver, gall bladder, and pancreas. The ultimate function of the gut is to break down foods and allow the nutrients to be distributed and used throughout the body to provide the energy and protection the body needs to survive.

GUT-MICROBIOME-BRAIN (GMB) CONNECTION. A network that links different systems of the body—including the central nervous, endocrine, metabolic, and immune systems—with bacteria in the *gut*, enabling your body to function properly. See also *gut*; *microbiome*.

HARDENING OF THE ARTERIES. See *atherosclerosis*.

HDL CHOLESTEROL. See *cholesterol*.

HEART ATTACK. A blockage of the blood supply to the heart, preventing a section of the heart from receiving adequate oxygen. Heart attacks usually occur when *plaque* deposits on the lining of the blood vessels rupture (break open), causing a blockage.

HEMATOCRIT. The ratio of the volume of *red blood cells* to the total volume of the liquid part of the blood.

HEMOGLOBIN. The protein in *red blood cells* that carries oxygen to the body's organs and tissues and transports the waste product carbon dioxide from the organs and tissues back to the lungs.

HEMOGLOBIN A1C TEST. A measure of *blood glucose* over time—for the last two or three months.

HEMORRHAGIC STROKE. See *stroke*.

HIGH BLOOD PRESSURE. See *hypertension*.

HIGH-DENSITY LIPOPROTEIN. See *cholesterol*.

HORMONES. The body's chemical messengers. Hormones travel through the bloodstream to tissues and organs, where they affect many processes, including growth and development, metabolism, sexual function, immune system function, reproduction, and mood.

HYPERTENSION. Also called high blood pressure, a common condition in which the long-term force of the blood against the *artery* walls is high enough to eventually cause health problems, such as heart disease. There are two types of hypertension. Primary hypertension develops gradually over the years and is caused by genetic and environmental factors, such as age, family history, lack of exercise, and *obesity*. Secondary hypertension is usually caused by an underlying health condition such as kidney disease or by the use of certain drugs.

HYPOTHYROIDISM. A condition in which your thyroid gland doesn't produce enough of certain critical hormones. It is also called underactive thyroid.

IMPLICIT BIAS. An unconscious belief or attitude toward a group, such as African Americans, that causes people to attribute certain behaviors or characteristics to all members of that group.

INCOMPLETE PROTEIN. A food that does not contain all nine of the essential *amino acids* that your body must get from your diet.

INSULIN. A *hormone* produced by the pancreas that is released into the blood when *glucose* levels rise. Insulin signals the cells to take in the glucose so that it can be be converted into energy for the body's use.

INSULIN RESISTANCE. A condition in which the cells stop responding normally to *insulin*, causing blood sugar levels to rise.

INSULIN-DEPENDENT DIABETES. See *type 1 diabetes.*

ISCHEMIC STROKE. See *stroke.*

JUVENILE DIABETES. See *type 1 diabetes.*

KETONES. Water-soluble molecules formed from fatty acids when the body doesn't produce enough *insulin* to convert *glucose* into energy. The body then burns ketones (fat) for energy instead of glucose.

LACTO VEGETARIAN DIET. A vegetarian diet that excludes meat, fish, poultry, and eggs, but allows dairy products.

LACTO-OVO VEGETARIAN DIET. A vegetarian diet that excludes meat, fish, and poultry, but allows dairy products and eggs.

LDL CHOLESTEROL. See *cholesterol.*

LEPTIN. A *hormone* predominantly made by fat (adipose) tissue that communicates with the brain to control appetite.

LEUKOPLAKIA. A condition that causes white patches to develop on the gums, the insides of the cheeks, the bottom of the mouth, and sometimes the tongue. These patches cannot be scraped off. Although doctors don't know what causes leukoplakia, they consider mouth irritants such as smoking to be the main culprit.

LIPID PEROXIDATION. Damage caused by *free radicals* to cellular membranes and other molecules in the cells that contain lipids (fats). This affects membrane permeability, nutrient transport, cellular signaling, and a variety of other cell functions, eventually leading to cell death.

LOW-DENSITY LIPOPROTEIN. See *cholesterol*.

MALIGNANT TUMOR. A cancerous tumor that develops when cells grow uncontrollably. These tumors can grow quickly and spread (metastasize) to other parts of the body.

MAMMOGRAM. An x-ray picture of the human breast used to identify breast cancer, usually through detection of characteristic masses and abnormal patterns of calcium deposits.

METABOLIC SYNDROME. A group of disorders that include high *blood pressure (hypertension)*, elevated blood sugar, high *cholesterol*, and excess body weight around the waist. Metabolic syndrome is a precursor to *diabetes* and is also strongly associated with heart disease and *stroke*.

METABOLISM. Chemical reactions in the body's cells that change the food we eat into the energy needed to fuel all body functions.

MICROBIOME. The microorganisms in a particular environment—including a part of the body, such as the *gut*—that include different types of bacteria. While bacteria are found throughout the gut, the highest concentration is found in the large intestine. These bacteria are responsible for a number of functions, including breaking down foods into basic components, synthesizing some vitamins, regulating metabolism, supporting the immune system, and more.

MITOCHONDRIA. Organelles (specialized cellular parts) within the cells that generate most of the chemical energy needed to fuel the cell's biochemical reactions.

MYCOTOXINS. Naturally occurring toxins that are produced by certain molds and are capable of causing disease and even death. Molds generally grow in dark, damp places.

NEPHRON. A functional unit of the kidney that filters the blood; reabsorbs some substances, such as *glucose*; and excretes excess water, salt, and nitrogenous waste in the form of urine.

NEUROTOXINS. Toxins that are destructive to nerve tissue.

OBESITY. An abnormal or excessive fat accumulation that presents a risk to health. A *body mass index (BMI)* over 30 indicates that a person is obese.

OFF-GASSING. The emission of *volatile organic compounds (VOCs)* from manufactured items such as paint, insulation, and carpets.

OMEGA-3 FATTY ACIDS. A class of essential fatty acids found in fish oils, especially oils from cold-water fish such as salmon, that act to lower the levels of *cholesterol*—including "bad" LDL (low-density lipoprotein) cholesterol—in the blood.

OPPORTUNISTIC BACTERIA. Bacteria that take advantage of certain opportunities, such as a weakened immune system, to cause disease.

ORAL THRUSH. Also called candidiasis or simply thrush, a yeast infection that develops inside the mouth, causing white or yellow bumps to form on the inner cheeks and tongue. Although this is most common in infants and toddlers, it can also occur in adults, with symptoms that include soreness or burning in the mouth; a cotton-like sensation in the mouth; dry, cracked skin at the corners of the mouth; and a bad taste.

OVO-VEGETARIAN DIET. A vegetarian diet that excludes meat, poultry, seafood, and dairy products, but allows eggs.

PAP TEST. Also known as a pap smear, a test that involves collecting cells from the cervix (the lower end of the uterus) to detect cervical cancer. A pap test can also detect human papillomavirus (HPV).

PERIODONTAL DISEASE. Also known as gum disease, inflammatory conditions that affect the tissues and bone which surround and support the teeth. Its earliest stage is known as *gingivitis,* and its more serious form is called *periodontitis.*

PERIODONTITIS. Severe gum disease that damages the gums and, without treatment, can harm the bone and connective tissue around the teeth. If left untreated, it can lead to loosening of the teeth and tooth loss.

PHTHALATES. A family of industrial chemicals that are used to make plastic more flexible and harder to break and are also used as solvents in cosmetics and other consumer products. Some of the health disorders associated with phthalates include asthma, attention-deficit hyperactivity disorder (ADHD), autism, low IQ, breast cancer, *obesity*, type 2 *diabetes*, and male fertility issues.

PHYTOCHEMICALS. Natural chemicals found in plants—fruits, vegetables, whole grains, nuts, seeds, and legumes—that contribute to their color, taste, and smell, and are thought to be largely responsible for the protective health benefits conferred by these plants.

PLAQUE. Deposits made up of *cholesterol*, fatty substances, cellular waste products, calcium, and fibrin (a clotting material) that form on the lining of *arteries*, thickening the arteries and slowing blood flow. Also, a soft, sticky film that builds up on the teeth. Containing millions of bacteria, dental plaque can cause tooth decay and gum disease if it is not removed through brushing and flossing.

POLLUTION INEQUITY. The concept that more vulnerable individuals, communities, and subpopulations—such as African Americans—are more likely to be exposed to higher levels of environmental pollution.

POLYCYSTIC KIDNEY DISEASE. An inherited disorder in which clusters of fluid-filled cysts develop within the kidneys, causing the kidneys to enlarge and lose function over time.

PREDIABETES. Also called borderline diabetes, a condition in which blood sugar levels are higher than normal but are not in the *diabetes* range.

PRIMARY HYPERTENSION. See *hypertension*.

PROBIOTIC FOODS. Foods containing healthful live *bacteria* that can directly benefit your *microbiome*. These foods include fermented pickles, sauerkraut, cheese, kimchi (spicy pickled cabbage), kombucha tea, natto, tempeh, traditional buttermilk, yogurt, and kefir.

PROBIOTIC SUPPLEMENTS. Supplements that provide beneficial *bacteria* in the form of tablets, powders, or capsules.

PSA (PROSTATE-SPECIFIC ANTIGEN) TEST. A blood test used to detect prostate cancer at an early stage.

RED BLOOD CELLS. The cells in blood that contain the protein *hemoglobin*, which permits the cells to transport oxygen throughout the body and remove the waste product carbon dioxide.

RENAL TUBULES. A series of tubes in the kidneys that reabsorb water, sodium, and *glucose* and return them to the blood.

RENIN-ANGIOTENSIN-ALDOSTERONE SYSTEM (RAAS). A *hormone* system that regulates *blood pressure* and fluid balance.

SECONDARY HYPERTENSION. See *hypertension*.

SENESCENCE. The process through which cells age, deteriorate in function, and permanently stop dividing, but do not die.

SICK BUILDING SYNDROME. A situation in which a building's occupants experience symptoms of ill health that appear to be associated with time spent in the building and not with a specific disease. Symptoms can include headaches, sinus problems, runny and irritated eyes and nose, throat irritation and tightness, fatigue, dizziness, and nausea.

SICKLE CELL ANEMIA. An inherited disease in which the *red blood cells* (RBCs) become misshapen, taking on a sickle or crescent shape, and also become less flexible, rendering them unable to carry sufficient oxygen and to pass easily through small *capillaries*. The sickle-shaped RBCs block the blood vessels and decrease blood flow, preventing needed oxygen and nutrients from reaching the body's tissues. This disorder is also known as sickle cell disease.

SICKLE CELL RETINOPATHY. A complication of *sickle cell anemia* in which sickle cells block the blood vessels in the retina and choroid of the eye, causing a thinning of the retina and abnormal blood vessel growth.

SIMPLE CARBOHYDRATES. Chemically simple carbohydrates, such as table sugar, that are broken down quickly by the body to be used as energy. See also *complex carbohydrates.*

STEM CELLS. A special type of cell, found in bone marrow and other tissues, that can develop into cells with specialized functions.

STRESS. The body's natural response to a potentially dangerous situation, whether real or imagined. Stress can result in a range of symptoms, including a racing heart, a surge of energy, increased *blood pressure*, nausea, and queasiness.

STROKE. An interruption or reduction of the blood supply to the brain that prevents oxygen and nutrients from reaching the brain. There are three types of strokes. An ischemic stroke occurs when a blood clot prevents blood from getting to the brain. A hemorrhagic stroke occurs when a weakened blood vessel bursts and bleeds into the surrounding brain. A transient ischemic attack, or TIA, occurs when the blood supply to an area of the brain is blocked but then restored.

SYSTOLIC PRESSURE. The force exerted by blood on *artery* walls resulting from contraction/pumping of the heart.

TARTAR. Also called calculus, a yellow- or brown-colored deposit that forms when *plaque* is allowed to harden on your teeth. Because tartar is strongly bonded to the tooth enamel, it can be removed only by a dental professional.

TELOMERES. Sections of DNA that sit at the end of the chromosomes in cells, much as protective plastic tips sit at the end of shoelaces. Telomeres stop the ends of chromosomes from fraying or sticking to each other and also play an important role in ensuring that DNA gets copied properly when cells divide.

THRUSH. See *oral thrush*.

TRANSIENT ISCHEMIC ATTACK (TIA). See *stroke*.

TRIGLYCERIDES. A type of lipid (fat) that makes up the bulk of fat cells and is released when the body needs energy.

TYPE 1 DIABETES. Also called juevenile diabetes and insulin-dependent diabetes, a genetic condition in which the pancreas secretes little or no *insulin*, causing blood sugar levels to be too high.

TYPE 2 DIABETES. A lifestyle-related condition in which the cells slowly decrease their response to normal levels of *insulin* or the body doesn't produce adequate insulin, causing blood sugar levels to be too high.

UNDERACTIVE THYROID. See *hypothyroidism*.

VASODILATORS. Medications that open (dilate) blood vessels, allowing blood to flow more easily through the blood vessels.

VASO-OCCLUSIVE CRISIS (VOC). A complication of *sickle cell anemia* that occurs when the sickled cells start clumping together and block the *capillaries*. VOCs can be extremely painful and, because of the blockage of blood vessels, can cause *stroke* and other serious problems.

VEGAN DIET. A vegetarian diet that excludes all animal products, including meat, fish, poultry, eggs, dairy, and even honey.

VEINS. Blood vessels that carry blood from the tissues of the body to the lungs and the heart.

VOLATILE ORGANIC COMPOUNDS (VOCS). Gases that are emitted into the air from products or processes. Some are harmful by themselves, including some that cause cancer, and some can react with other gases to form harmful substances.

WHITE BLOOD CELLS. Also called leukocytes, the cells in blood that are involved in protecting the body against infectious disease and foreign invaders. There are several types of white blood cells, including lymphocytes, monocytes, neutrophils, basophils, and eosinophils.

A Guide to Dietary Supplements

Choosing a nutritional supplement can be intimidating. In recent years, the number and variety of supplements on store shelves have exploded, making the process of purchasing the right product for you even more confusing. But a trip to the supplements aisle doesn't have to be frustrating. This section provides guidance in purchasing and using dietary supplements that will help you home in on the best products for your personal health plan.

BUY PHARMACEUTICAL GRADE OR WHOLE FOOD-BASED SUPPLEMENTS

Whenever possible, buy pharmaceutical-grade supplements, which must exceed 99-percent purity and not contain any fillers, binders, or other inactive ingredients. Pharmaceutical-grade supplements are also highly bioavailable, meaning that your body can more easily absorb and use the nutrients they provide. Unfortunately, these supplements are difficult to find and often must be ordered. When pharmaceutical-grade supplements are simply not available, choose whole food-based products, which are sourced from actual food and therefore contain numerous additional compounds that support bioavailability. Whether the supplement is whole food-based or not, always read the label on the bottle to determine if the product contains any ingredients that may cause an allergic reaction, such as soy, dairy, or gluten. Finally, make sure that the supplement provides the specific form recommended in this book—for instance, be certain you have vitamin D_3 and not vitamin D$_2$—and check the dosage so that you'll be able to easily take the recommended amount.

If you want further guidance in choosing supplement brands, visit ConsumerLab.com. This nonprofit independent organization tests different brands of supplements and determines which ones contain what their labels say they contain and also offer the best price. It costs a few dollars a month to access the information on this website, but in the end, the information may save you money by helping you find good-quality products.

PROCESSING AND PACKAGING

The manner in which supplements are both processed and packaged has a significant effect on their nutritional impact. In the same way that overcooking a food destroys its nutrients, the strength of a supplement is diminished if it is heated beyond 125°F during processing. Whenever possible, look for a supplement that has been freeze-dried or processed at a low temperature. In addition to the effect of heat on supplements, exposure to light and air also diminishes their effectiveness. Dark plastic bottles do a better job of blocking light than do the typical white plastic bottles, but dark amber or dark blue glass bottles are the best choice. Also, always check that the bottle has been vacuum-sealed, which not only ensures that the product is fresh but also prevents anyone from tampering with its contents.

DOSAGE

You may be wondering why dosages for some of the supplements listed in this book are higher than the daily amounts recommended by the Food and Drug Administration. The answer is that the FDA's recommendations are merely designed to ward off conditions caused by nutritional insufficiencies. They are not intended to prevent or alleviate the diseases plaguing our modern lives. For example, a dose of 60 mg of vitamin C per day, as suggested by the FDA, will help you avoid scurvy, an illness caused by vitamin C deficiency. It will not, however, decrease your risk of cancer, which, according to some studies, may be lowered by taking 300 mg of vitamin C per day. Similarly, while the FDA urges people to get 400 IU of vitamin D every day, diabetics have a much better chance of improving their insulin sensitivity by taking between 2,000 and 5,000 IU on a daily basis, to name but one of the positive effects of elevated vitamin D dosage.

In many instances, the FDA's recommendations are appropriate, and you should always be careful not to take any supplement in an amount that might result in toxicity. More and more, however, research is proving the advantages of exceeding the typical dosage of certain supplements. While this book provides you with detailed information on supplement quantities, you should speak to your doctor for further advice on the subject, especially if you are taking prescription medications for any disorder.

USING THE TABLE OF SUPPLEMENT RECOMMENDATIONS

In addition to a comprehensive multivitamin for overall wellness, I recommend the nutritional supplements listed in the following table to treat the specific illnesses and conditions discussed in this book, as well as for better health. Each supplement offers significant benefits that are supported by research. Please note that in the chapter on each disorder, I recommend the most important supplements in the treatment of that disorder—those that have been proven to have the greatest benefits. In the following table, for each disorder, I have listed all of those important supplements. I have also included additional supplements that can be helpful. Start by taking the supplements highlighted in the chapter on the disorder, and if you feel you need more nutritional support, begin adding the other supplements listed in the table. There is no reason to overdo supplementation. Listen closely to your body and take only what it truly needs.

Note that in addition to recommending nutritional supplements for the treatment of the disorders and conditions discussed in this book, in the last few pages of the table, I recommend supplements that can help enhance men's health and women's health. Consider these supplements when putting together your supplement regimen.

Finally, unless otherwise directed, take supplements with a meal rather than on an empty stomach. When you consume foods, it starts a series of digestive processes that help the body absorb the nutrients in the food. These processes will also optimize the absorption of nutritional supplements. In addition, taking supplements with food can help prevent the stomach upset some people experience when using these products on an empty stomach.

Supplement Recommendations for Medical Conditions and Better Health		
AGING		
SUPPLEMENT	DOSAGE	CONSIDERATIONS
Alpha-Lipoic Acid	100 to 200 mg three times daily.	If you suffer from thyroid disease, diabetes, or vitamin B_1 deficiency, use alcohol excessively, or are undergoing cancer treatment, talk to your doctor before taking alpha-lipoic acid supplements. Avoid supplementation if you are pregnant or breastfeeding.
Astaxanthin	Follow the manufacturer's instructions.	Avoid supplementation if you are pregnant or breastfeeding.
Blueberry Extract	Follow the manufacturer's instructions.	If you suffer from diabetes, talk to your doctor before taking blueberry extract supplements. Avoid supplementation if you are pregnant or breastfeeding.
Curcumin (Bio-Curcumin) Extract (Turmeric)	250 mg twice daily on an empty stomach.	Avoid supplementation if you are pregnant or breastfeeding, or suffer from gallbladder problems. Stop taking curcumin at least two weeks before any scheduled surgery.
Grape Seed Extract (95 percent OPC)	50 to 200 mg once daily.	Avoid supplementation if you are pregnant or breastfeeding.

N-Acetyl Cysteine (NAC)	600 mg once daily.	If you suffer from asthma, talk to your doctor before taking NAC supplements. Avoid supplementation if you are pregnant or breastfeeding unless absolutely needed. Avoid supplementation if you have an allergy to acetyl cysteine.
Omega-3 Fatty Acids	1,000 mg once daily with food.	If you have problems with your blood pressure, talk to your doctor before taking omega-3 fatty acid supplements.
Pomegranate Extract	250 to 500 mg once daily.	If you are pregnant or breastfeeding, or using any medications, talk to your doctor before taking pomegranate extract. Stop taking pomegranate extract at least two weeks before any scheduled surgery.
Probiotics	Choose a product that provides at least five different types of bacteria and more than 70 billion colonies, and follow the manufacturer's instructions.	If you take immune suppression drugs, are undergoing treatment for a fungal infection, have a weak immune system, or have been diagnosed with pancreatitis, do not take probiotic supplements.
Quercetin	500 mg twice daily.	Higher dosages may cause kidney damage. Possible side effects include headaches and tingling of the arms and legs. Avoid supplementation if you are pregnant or breastfeeding.
Resveratrol	20 to 40 mg once daily.	Store supplements in a cool, dry place. Avoid supplementation if you are pregnant or breastfeeding, or suffer from a hormone-sensitive condition, such as breast cancer, uterine cancer, ovarian cancer, endometriosis, or uterine fibroids. Stop taking resveratrol at least two weeks before any scheduled surgery.

Selenium	200 mcg once daily for adults, 60 mcg once daily for women who are pregnant, 70 mcg once daily for women who are breastfeeding.	If you suffer from thyroid disease, have a family history of prostate cancer, or are using proton-pump inhibitors or histamine blockers, talk to your doctor before taking selenium supplements. Possible side effects include reduced fertility in men.
Superoxide Dismutase (SOD)	150 mg once daily.	Not enough is known about the use of superoxide dismutase during pregnancy and breastfeeding. Stay on the safe side and avoid use.
Vitamin C	300 mg once daily for adults, 60 mg once daily for women who are pregnant or breastfeeding.	Higher dosages may cause kidney stones and severe diarrhea. Avoid supplementation if you suffer from sickle cell disease, cancer, hemochromatosis, diabetes, glucose-6-phosphate dehydrogenase (G6PD), or are scheduled for a heart procedure.
Zinc Citrate or Picolinate	15 to 25 mg once daily.	Avoid taking zinc at the same time as calcium, copper, iron, or soy, as it can interfere with the absorption of these nutrients. Zinc supplements can also decrease the absorption of the antibiotics fluoroquinolone and tetracycline.

CANCER		
SUPPLEMENT	DOSAGE	CONSIDERATIONS
Alpha-Lipoic Acid	100 to 200 mg three times daily.	If you suffer from thyroid disease, diabetes, or vitamin B_1 deficiency, use alcohol excessively, or are undergoing cancer treatment, talk to your doctor before taking alpha-lipoic acid supplements. Avoid supplementation if you are pregnant or breastfeeding.

Andrographis	400 mg twice daily for no more than fourteen days at a time.	If you are undergoing cancer treatment, talk to your doctor before taking Andrographis supplements. Avoid supplementation if you are pregnant or breastfeeding, have fertility problems, or suffer from an autoimmune disease, such as multiple sclerosis, lupus, or rheumatoid arthritis.
Astaxanthin	Follow the manufacturer's instructions.	Avoid supplementation if you are pregnant or breastfeeding.
Black Raspberry Extract	Follow the manufacturer's instructions.	Avoid supplementation if you are pregnant or breastfeeding.
Blueberry Extract	Follow the manufacturer's instructions.	Talk to your doctor before taking blueberry extract supplements. Avoid supplementation if you are pregnant or breastfeeding.
Curcumin (Bio-Curcumin) Extract (Turmeric)	50 to 100 mg once daily on an empty stomach.	Avoid supplementation if you are pregnant or breastfeeding, have gallbladder problems, or are undergoing chemotherapy. Stop taking curcumin at least two weeks before any scheduled surgery.
Echinacea	250 to 500 mg for no more than eight weeks at a time.	If you are undergoing cancer treatment, talk to your doctor before taking echinacea supplements. Possible side effects include dizziness and nausea. Avoid supplementation if you are pregnant or breastfeeding; have allergies; or suffer from an autoimmune disease, such as multiple sclerosis, lupus, or rheumatoid arthritis.
Elderberry Extract	Follow the manufacturer's instructions.	Avoid supplementation if you are pregnant or breastfeeding, or suffer from an autoimmune disease, such as multiple sclerosis, lupus, or rheumatoid arthritis.

Grape Seed Extract (95 percent OPC)	50 to 200 mg once daily.	Avoid supplementation if you are pregnant or breastfeeding.
Green Tea Extract	6 to 9 drops added to 32 ounces of water to be ingested throughout the day.	If you suffer from diabetes, osteoporosis, or glaucoma, talk to your doctor before taking green tea extract. Avoid supplementation if you suffer from a bleeding disorder, anxiety disorder, anemia, heart problems, or liver disease.
N-Acetyl Cysteine (NAC)	600 mg once daily.	If you suffer from asthma, talk to your doctor before taking NAC supplements. Avoid supplementation if you are pregnant or breastfeeding unless absolutely needed. Avoid supplementation if you have an allergy to acetyl cysteine.
Olive Leaf Extract	500 mg twice daily with food.	Avoid supplementation if you are pregnant or breastfeeding.
Omega-3 Fatty Acids	1 to 3 g once daily.	If you have problems with your blood pressure, talk to your doctor before taking omega-3 fatty acid supplements.
Pomegranate Extract	250 to 500 mg once daily.	If you are pregnant or breastfeeding, or using any medications, talk to your doctor before taking pomegranate extract. Stop taking pomegranate extract at least two weeks before any scheduled surgery.
Probiotics	Choose a product that provides at least five different types of bacteria and more than 70 billion colonies, and follow the manufacturer's instructions.	If you take immune suppression drugs, are undergoing treatment for a fungal infection, have a weak immune system, or have been diagnosed with pancreatitis, do not take probiotic supplements.

Quercetin	500 mg twice daily.	Higher dosages may cause kidney damage. Possible side effects include headaches and tingling of the arms and legs. Avoid supplementation if you are pregnant or breastfeeding.
Resveratrol	20 to 40 mg once daily.	Store supplements in a cool, dry place. Avoid supplementation if you are pregnant or breastfeeding, or suffer from a hormone-sensitive condition, such as breast cancer, uterine cancer, ovarian cancer, endometriosis, or uterine fibroids. Stop taking resveratrol at least two weeks before any scheduled surgery.
Selenium	200 mcg once daily for adults, 60 mcg once daily for women who are pregnant, 70 mcg once daily for women who are breastfeeding.	If you suffer from thyroid disease, have a family history of prostate cancer, or are using proton-pump inhibitors or histamine blockers, talk to your doctor before taking selenium supplements. Possible side effects include reduced fertility in men.
Vitamin C	300 mg once daily for adults, 60 mg once daily for women who are pregnant or breastfeeding.	Higher dosages may cause kidney stones and severe diarrhea. Avoid supplementation if you suffer from sickle cell disease, cancer, hemochromatosis, diabetes, or glucose-6-phosphate dehydrogenase (G6PD), or are scheduled for a heart procedure.
Vitamin D_3	5,000 IU once daily.	Get a 25-OH vitamin D test or talk to your doctor before taking vitamin D_3 supplements at levels above 1,000 IU daily.
Vitamin K_2	70 to 80 mcg once daily for men, 55 to 65 mcg once daily for women.	If you suffer from kidney or liver disease, talk to your doctor before taking vitamin K_2 supplements.

Zinc Citrate or Picolinate	15 to 25 mg once daily.	Avoid taking zinc at the same time as calcium, copper, iron, or soy, as it can interfere with the absorption of these nutrients. Zinc can also decrease absorption of antibiotics fluoroquinolone and tetracycline.
CARDIOVASCULAR DISEASE		
SUPPLEMENT	DOSAGE	CONSIDERATIONS
Aged Garlic Extract	500 to 600 mg three times daily.	If you are on blood thinners or have a bleeding disorder, talk to your doctor before taking aged garlic extract supplements. Possible side effects include gastrointestinal irritation. Avoid supplementation if you are pregnant or breastfeeding. Stop taking aged garlic extract at least two weeks before any scheduled surgery.
Coenzyme Q$_{10}$ (Ubiquinol)	100 mg one to three times daily with food.	If you have problems with blood pressure, talk to your doctor before taking coenzyme Q$_{10}$ supplements. Avoid supplementation if you are pregnant or breastfeeding. Stop taking coenzyme Q$_{10}$ at least two weeks before any scheduled surgery.
Dark Chocolate (85 to 99 Percent Cacao)	50 to 100 g daily.	Due to the caffeine content of chocolate, do not eat any more than this amount if you are pregnant or breastfeeding. Possible side effects include anxiety, migraine headaches, increased heart rate, and stomach disturbances. Stop eating dark chocolate at least two weeks before any scheduled surgery.
Grape Seed Extract (95 percent OPC)	50 to 200 mg once daily.	Avoid supplementation if you are pregnant or breastfeeding.
Hawthorn Berry Extract	160 to 450 mg once or twice daily.	If you are using medications to treat heart disease, talk to your doctor before taking hawthorn berry extract supplements. Avoid supplementation if you are pregnant or breastfeeding.

L-Arginine	1,000 mg once to three times daily.	Possible side effects include diarrhea, nausea, and tightness in the chest. Avoid supplementation if you are pregnant or breastfeeding; suffer from low blood pressure, herpes, asthma, or allergies; or have had a heart attack. Stop taking L-arginine at least two weeks before any scheduled surgery.
L-Carnitine	500 to 1,000 mg twice daily before 3:00 PM.	If you have experienced seizures or suffer from thyroid disease, talk to your doctor before taking L-carnitine supplements.
Lycopene	5 to 20 mg once daily.	Avoid supplementation if you are pregnant or breastfeeding, or have been diagnosed with prostate cancer.
Magnesium Citrate or Glycinate	400 to 800 mg once daily.	Some people experience diarrhea at levels of 600 mg daily and should take less than this amount.
Natto kinase	Follow the manufacturer's instructions.	Avoid supplementation if you are pregnant or breastfeeding, or suffer from a bleeding disorder. Stop taking natto kinase at least two weeks before any scheduled surgery.
Omega-3 Fatty Acids	1,000 to 2,000 mg once daily with food.	If you have problems with your blood pressure, talk to your doctor before taking omega-3 fatty acid supplements.
Pomegranate Extract	250 to 500 mg once daily.	If you are pregnant or breastfeeding, or using any medications, talk to your doctor before taking pomegranate extract. Stop taking pomegranate extract at least two weeks before any scheduled surgery.
Vitamin B Complex	15 mg of B_3, 2 mg of B_6, 400 mcg of B_9, and 2.4 mcg of B_{12} once daily.	If you have low blood pressure, stomach ulcers, or diabetes, or suffer from kidney, liver, gallbladder, or heart disease, talk to your doctor before taking vitamin B_3 supplements. Avoid supplementation with vitamin B_{12} if you are allergic to cobalt or cobalamin, or suffer from Leber's disease.

Vitamin D$_3$	2,000 to 5,000 IU once daily.	Get a 25-OH vitamin D test or talk to your doctor before taking vitamin D$_3$ supplements at levels above 1,000 IU daily.

DIABETES, TYPE 2		
SUPPLEMENT	**DOSAGE**	**CONSIDERATIONS**
Alpha-Lipoic Acid	100 to 200 mg three times daily.	If you suffer from thyroid disease, diabetes, or vitamin B$_1$ deficiency, use alcohol excessively, or are undergoing cancer treatment, talk to your doctor before taking alpha-lipoic acid supplements. Avoid supplementation if you are pregnant or breastfeeding. This supplement works best when taken with 400 to 600 mg gamma-linolenic acid (GLA).
Chromium Picolinate	1,000 mcg once daily.	Higher dosages to treat specific diseases should be discussed with your doctor. Avoid supplementation if you suffer from diabetes, liver or kidney disease, behavioral or psychiatric conditions, chromate or leather allergies, or are pregnant or breastfeeding.
Cinnulin PF (Cinnamon Extract)	125 to 150 mg three times daily.	If you suffer from diabetes, talk to your doctor before taking cinnulin PF supplements. Avoid supplementation if you are pregnant or breast feeding or suffer from liver disease. Stop taking cinnulin PF at least two weeks before any scheduled surgery.
Coenzyme Q$_{10}$ (Ubiquinol)	100 mg one to three times daily with food.	If you have problems with your blood pressure, talk to your doctor before taking coenzyme Q$_{10}$ supplements. Avoid supplementation if you are pregnant or breastfeeding. Stop taking coenzyme Q$_{10}$ at least two weeks before any scheduled surgery.

DHEA	50 to 100 mg once daily for men, 25 mg once daily for women. Get your DHEA level checked by your doctor for a personalized dosage.	Avoid supplementation if you are pregnant or breastfeeding, or suffer from liver problems, polycystic ovary syndrome, or a hormone-sensitive condition, such as breast cancer, uterine cancer, ovarian cancer, endometriosis, uterine fibroids, or prostate cancer. If you suffer from diabetes, mood disorder, or cholesterol problems, talk to your doctor before taking DHEA supplements.
Green Tea Extract	6 to 9 drops added to 32 ounces of water to be ingested throughout the day.	If you suffer from diabetes, osteoporosis, or glaucoma, talk to your doctor before taking green tea extract supplements. Avoid supplementation if you suffer from a bleeding disorder, anxiety disorder, anemia, heart problems, or liver disease.
Gymnema Silvestre	Follow the manufacturer's instructions.	If you suffer from diabetes, talk to your doctor before taking gymnema silvestre supplements. Its use is to reduce cravings for sweets. Avoid supplementation if you are pregnant or breastfeeding. Stop taking gymnema silvestre at least two weeks before any scheduled surgery.
Vitamin D_3	2,000 to 5,000 IU once daily.	Get a 25-OH vitamin D test and talk to your doctor before taking vitamin D_3 supplements at levels above 1,000 IU daily.
GUT-MICROBIOME-BRAIN HEALTH		
SUPPLEMENT	**DOSAGE**	**CONSIDERATIONS**
Probiotics	Choose a product that provides at least five different types of bacteria and more than 70 billion colonies, and follow the manufacturer's instructions.	If you take immune suppression drugs, are undergoing treatment for a fungal infection, have a weak immune system, or have been diagnosed with pancreatitis, do not take probiotic supplements.

HYPERTENSION		
SUPPLEMENT	DOSAGE	CONSIDERATIONS
Aged Garlic Extract	500 to 600 mg three times daily.	If you are on blood thinners or have a bleeding disorder, talk to your doctor before taking aged garlic extract supplements. Possible side effects include gastrointestinal irritation. Avoid supplementation if you are pregnant or breastfeeding. Stop taking aged garlic extract at least two weeks before any scheduled surgery.
Coenzyme Q_{10} (Ubiquinol)	100 mg one to three times daily with food.	If you have problems with your blood pressure, talk to your doctor before taking coenzyme Q_{10} supplements. Avoid supplementation if you are pregnant or breastfeeding. Stop taking coenzyme Q_{10} at least two weeks before any scheduled surgery.
Dark Chocolate (85 to 99 Percent Cacao)	50 to 100 g daily.	Due to the caffeine content of chocolate, do not eat more than this amount if you are pregnant or breastfeeding. Possible side effects include anxiety, migraine headaches, increased heart rate, and stomach disturbances. Stop eating dark chocolate at least two weeks before any scheduled surgery.
Folic Acid (Vitamin B_9)	400 to 500 mcg once daily.	Doses of folic acid greater than 1 mg daily may cause headache, diarrhea, rash, nausea, stomach upset, behavior changes, gas, and other side effects.
Grape Seed Extract (95 Percent OPC)	50 to 200 mg once daily.	Avoid supplementation if you are pregnant or breastfeeding.
Hawthorn Berry Extract	160 to 900 mg once or twice daily.	If you are using medications to treat heart disease, talk to your doctor before taking hawthorn berry extract supplements. Avoid supplementation if you are pregnant or breastfeeding.

L-Arginine	1,000 mg once to three times daily.	Possible side effects include diarrhea, nausea, and tightness in the chest. Avoid supplementation if you are pregnant or breastfeeding, suffer from low blood pressure, herpes, asthma, or allergies, or have had a heart attack. Stop taking L-arginine at least two weeks before any scheduled surgery.
Lycopene	5 to 20 mg once daily.	Avoid supplementation if you are pregnant or breastfeeding or have been diagnosed with prostate cancer.
Magnesium Citrate or Glycinate	400 to 500 mg time-released formula once daily.	Some people experience diarrhea at levels of 600 mg daily and should take less than this amount.
Natto kinase	Follow the manufacturer's instructions.	Avoid supplementation if you are pregnant or breastfeeding, or suffer from a bleeding disorder. Stop taking natto kinase at least two weeks before any scheduled surgery.
Olive Leaf Extract	500 mg twice daily with food.	Avoid supplementation if you are pregnant or breastfeeding.
Omega-3 Fatty Acids	1,000 mg once daily with food.	If you have problems with your blood pressure, talk to your doctor before taking omega-3 fatty acid supplements.
Pomegranate Extract	250 to 500 mg once daily.	If you are pregnant or breastfeeding or using any medications, talk to your doctor before taking pomegranate extract. Stop taking pomegranate extract at least two weeks before any scheduled surgery.
Vitamin D$_3$	2,000 to 5,000 IU once daily.	Get a 25-OH vitamin D test or talk to your doctor before taking vitamin D$_3$ supplements at levels above 1,000 IU daily.
Vitamin E (Mixed Tocopherols and Tocotrienols)	100 to 400 IU once daily.	If you are using blood thinners, talk to your doctor before taking vitamin E supplements.

Vitamin K$_2$	70 to 80 mcg once daily for men, 55 to 65 mcg once daily for women.	If you suffer from kidney or liver disease, talk to your doctor before taking vitamin K$_2$ supplements.

KIDNEY DISEASE		
SUPPLEMENT	**DOSAGE**	**CONSIDERATIONS**
DHEA	50 mg once daily for men, 25 mg once daily for women. Get your DHEA level checked by your doctor for a personalized dosage.	Avoid supplementation if you are pregnant or breastfeeding, or suffer from liver problems, polycystic ovary syndrome, or a hormone-sensitive condition, such as breast cancer, uterine cancer, ovarian cancer, endometriosis, uterine fibroids, or prostate cancer. If you suffer from diabetes, mood disorder, or cholesterol problems, talk to your doctor before taking DHEA supplements.
L-Theanine	50 to 200 mg once daily.	Avoid supplementation if you are pregnant or breastfeeding.
Vitamin D$_3$	2,000 to 5,000 IU once daily.	Get a 25-OH vitamin D test and talk to your doctor before taking vitamin D$_3$ supplements at levels above 1,000 IU daily.
Vitamin K$_2$	80 mcg once daily for men, 65 mcg once daily for women.	If you suffer from kidney or liver disease, talk to your doctor before taking vitamin K$_2$ supplements.

OBESITY		
SUPPLEMENT	**DOSAGE**	**CONSIDERATIONS**
5-Hydroxy-tryptophan (5-HTP)	50 mg twice to three times daily.	Possible side effects include heartburn, stomachache, nausea, vomiting, diarrhea, drowsiness, muscular problems, and sexual problems. Avoid supplementation if you are pregnant or breastfeeding; if you have Down syndrome; or if you are currently taking antidepressants.

Coenzyme Q$_{10}$ (Ubiquinol)	100 mg once to three times daily with food.	If you have problems with your blood pressure, talk to your doctor before taking coenzyme Q$_{10}$ supplements. Avoid supplementation if you are pregnant or breastfeeding. Stop taking coenzyme Q$_{10}$ at least two weeks before any scheduled surgery.
Glisodin	150 mg once or twice daily.	Talk to your doctor before taking glisodin supplements.
Glutathione	500 to 1,000 mg once daily.	Avoid supplementation if you are pregnant or breastfeeding.
Green Tea Extract	6 to 9 drops added to 32 ounces of water to be ingested throughout the day.	If you suffer from diabetes, osteoporosis, or glaucoma, talk to your doctor before taking green tea extract supplements. Avoid supplementation if you suffer from a bleeding disorder, anxiety disorder, anemia, heart problems, or liver disease.
Greens Powder	Follow the manufacturer's instructions.	Talk to your doctor before taking greens powder supplements.
Irvingia Gabonensis	150 mg twice daily.	Possible side effects include flatulence, headaches, and sleep problems. Avoid supplementation if you are pregnant or breastfeeding.
L-Theanine	100 mg three times daily.	Avoid supplementation if you are pregnant or breastfeeding.
N-Acetyl Cysteine (NAC)	1,000 mg once daily.	If you suffer from asthma, talk to your doctor before taking NAC supplements. Avoid supplementation if you are pregnant or breastfeeding unless absolutely needed. Avoid supplementation if you have an allergy to acetyl cysteine.
Reds Powder	Follow the manufacturer's instructions.	Talk to your doctor before taking reds powder supplements.

| Saffron | 30 mg twice daily. | Possible side effects include dry mouth, anxiety, dizziness, nausea, fatigue, headaches, and a change in appetite. Avoid supplementation if you are pregnant or breastfeeding, suffer from a bipolar disorder, or are allergic to the plant species Lolia, Olea, or Salsola. |
| Vitamin D₃ | 2,000 to 5,000 IU once daily. | Get a 25-OH vitamin D test and talk to your doctor before taking vitamin D₃ supplements at levels above 1,000 IU daily. |

SICKLE CELL DISEASE		
SUPPLEMENT	**DOSAGE**	**CONSIDERATIONS**
Folic Acid (Vitamin B₉)	1 mg once daily.	Doses of folic acid greater than 1 mg daily may cause headache, diarrhea, rash, nausea, stomach upset, behavior changes, gas, and other side effects. If you are treating a child, check the dosage with your child's doctor.
Omega-3 Fatty Acids	1,000 mg to 2,000 mg once daily with food.	If you have problems with your blood pressure, talk to your doctor before taking omega-3 fatty acid supplements.
Vitamin D₃	2,000 to 5,000 IU once daily.	Get a 25-OH vitamin D test and talk to your doctor before taking vitamin D₃ supplements at levels above 1,000 IU daily.

MEN'S HEALTH		
SUPPLEMENT	**DOSAGE**	**CONSIDERATIONS**
Beta-Sitosterol	20 to 40 mg three times daily.	Avoid supplementation if you suffer from sitosterolomia.
Diindolylmethane (DIM)	Follow the manufacturer's instructions.	Avoid supplementation if you suffer from a hormone-sensitive condition, such as prostate cancer.

Flax Lignans	10 to 30 mg once daily.	If you suffer from diabetes, gastrointestinal obstruction, or a hormone-sensitive condition such as prostate cancer, talk to your doctor before taking flax lignans. Avoid supplementation if you have high triglycerides or suffer from a bleeding disorder.
Green Tea Extract	6 to 9 drops added to 32 ounces of water to be ingested throughout the day.	If you suffer from diabetes, osteoporosis, or glaucoma, talk to your doctor before taking green tea extract. Avoid supplementation if you suffer from a bleeding disorder, anxiety disorder, anemia, heart problems, or liver disease.
HMR lignans	10 to 30 mg once daily.	If you suffer from diabetes, gastrointestinal obstruction, or a hormone-sensitive condition, such as prostate cancer, talk to your doctor before taking HMR lignans. Avoid supplementation if you have high triglycerides or suffer from a bleeding disorder.
Indole-3-Carbinol	200 to 400 mg once daily.	Higher dosages may cause balance problems, tremors, and nausea.
Lycopene	5 to 20 mg once daily.	Avoid supplementation if you have been diagnosed with prostate cancer.
Saw Palmetto	160 mg twice daily.	Possible side effects include dizziness, headaches, nausea, vomiting, constipation, and diarrhea. Stop taking saw palmetto at least two weeks before any scheduled surgery.
Selenium	200 mcg once daily.	If you suffer from thyroid disease, have a family history of prostate cancer, or are using proton-pump inhibitors or histamine blockers, talk to your doctor before taking selenium supplements. Possible side effects include reduced fertility in men.

Vitamin D₃	2,000 to 5,000 IU once daily.	Get a 25-OH vitamin D test and talk to your doctor before taking vitamin D₃ supplements at levels above 1,000 IU daily.
Zinc Citrate or Picolinate	15 to 25 mg once daily.	Avoid taking zinc at the same time as calcium, copper, iron, or soy, as it can interfere with the absorption of these nutrients. Zinc supplements can also decrease the absorption of the antibiotics fluoroquinolone and tetracycline.

WOMEN'S HEALTH		
SUPPLEMENT	**DOSAGE**	**CONSIDERATIONS**
Calcium	Daily calcium intake should be about 1,000 mg per day from both diet and supplementation.	Calcium supplements can decrease the absorption of aluminum, magnesium, zinc, iron, manganese, phosphorus, thyroid medication, and the antibiotics ciprofloxacin, fluoroquinolone, and tetracycline. Talk to your doctor before starting supplementation.
Diindolylmethane (DIM)	Follow the manufacturer's instructions.	Consult a physician before using if you are pregnant or breastfeeding, or suffer from a hormone-sensitive condition, such as breast cancer, uterine cancer, ovarian cancer, endometriosis, or uterine fibroids.
Flax Lignans	10 to 30 mg once daily.	If you suffer from diabetes, gastrointestinal obstruction, or a hormone-sensitive condition, such as breast cancer, uterine cancer, ovarian cancer, endometriosis, or uterine fibroids, talk to your doctor before taking flax lignans. Avoid supplementation if you are pregnant or breastfeeding, have high triglycerides, or suffer from a bleeding disorder.

Green Tea Extract	6 to 9 drops added to 32 ounces of water to be ingested throughout the day.	If you suffer from diabetes, osteoporosis, or glaucoma, talk to your doctor before taking green tea extract. Avoid supplementation if you suffer from a bleeding disorder, anxiety disorder, anemia, heart problems, or liver disease.
HMR lignans	10 to 30 mg once daily.	If you suffer from diabetes, gastrointestinal obstruction, or a hormone-sensitive condition, such as breast cancer, uterine cancer, ovarian cancer, endometriosis, or uterine fibroids, talk to your doctor before taking HMR lignans. Avoid supplementation if you are pregnant or breastfeeding, have high triglycerides, or suffer from a bleeding disorder.
Indole-3-Carbinol	200 to 400 mg once daily.	Higher doses may cause balance problems, tremors, and nausea. Avoid supplementation if you are pregnant or breastfeeding.
Lycopene	5 to 20 mg once daily.	Avoid supplementation if you are pregnant or breastfeeding.
Vitamin D$_3$	2,000 to 5,000 IU once daily.	Get a 25-OH vitamin D test and talk to your doctor before taking vitamin D$_3$ supplements at levels above 1,000 IU daily.

Resources

A number of organizations, websites, articles, and books can enhance your understanding of health conditions and related issues, and also guide you in implementing the suggestions that are offered throughout this book. To help you easily find what you are looking for, this resource list has been broken up into the following sections: *Black Health; General Health; Medication Information; Environmental Health and Air Quality; Nutrition and Supplements; Special Diets; Recipes;* and *Devices and Apps.* Although we've tried to make this resource list as user-friendly as possible, please be aware that there is a certain amount of overlap between some sections. For instance, you'll find guidance for following the Mediterranean Diet under the *Special Diets* section, but if you're looking for Mediterranean Diet recipes, you'll also want to check the *Recipes* section.

BLACK HEALTH

BLKHLTH (Black Health)
Website: www.blkhth.com
BLKHLTH critically engages and challenges racism and its impact on Black health. Essays focus on diverse topics, including food deserts, democracy, the Black Panthers, Black health, and the fight for health equity.

Black Health Matters
Website: https://blackhealthmatters.com
Unrelated to this book, the Black Health Matters website offers many helpful articles on health topics that are of particular interest to the Black

community, including vitamin D, diabetes, heart disease, sickle cell disease, and more.

EBONY Health

Website: www.ebony.com/health
This website of *EBONY* magazine provides articles on fighting injustice in health care, heart disease, the health battles of well-known African Americans, and other topics of interest.

GENERAL HEALTH

American Diabetes Association

Website: www.diabetes.org
The website of the American Diabetes Association presents a wealth of information on the different forms of diabetes, including information on treatment and care, and also provides easy-to-prepare diabetes-friendly recipes.

American Heart Association

Website: www.heart.org
The purpose of the American Heart Association is to help reduce disability and death from cardiovascular disease. The organization's website provides useful articles on heart disease and also includes a section on healthy living.

American Stroke Association

Website: www.stroke.org
The American Stroke Association, a division of the American Heart Association, offers information on stroke—its risk factors, symptoms, and treatment; support for caregivers and family members; and recommendations for heart-healthy eating, fitness, and other important lifestyle issues.

Cleveland Clinic

Website: https://my.clevelandclinic.org/search
The website of the Cleveland Clinic allows you to access excellent articles on coronary artery disease, diabetes, hypertension, and other health disorders.

Harvard Health Publishing

Website: www.health.harvard.edu

Provided by Harvard University, the Harvard Health Publishing website features excellent easy-to-understand information on hypertension, cardiovascular disease, diabetes, and other health disorders.

National Kidney Foundation
Website: www.kidney.org
Visit the National Kidney Foundation website for information on kidney "basics" and available treatments for kidney disease. Various means of support for patients and family are also offered.

Sickle Cell Disease Association Repository
Website: www.sicklecelldisease.net
The SCD repository website was designed to help you understand sickle cell disease risk factors, signs, symptoms, treatment options, and more.

WebMD
Website: www.webmd.com
WebMD is an excellent source of information on various health disorders—including those that concern many African Americans—as well as medications, supplements, healthy living, and other health-related topics.

MEDICATION INFORMATION

Drugs.com
Website: Drugs.com
A great resource for anyone who wants to know more about the medications they take, Drugs.com allows you to learn about prescription meds in their A-to-Z drugs list; become better informed about OTC meds through their over-the-counter drug database; learn more about side effects; use their Drug Interactions Checker to see if the meds that have been prescribed for you may cause problems when taken together; and explore medication options for health issues such as angina, diabetes, hypertension, and more.

ENVIRONMENTAL HEALTH AND AIR QUALITY

■ GENERAL INFORMATION

Body Burden: The Pollution in Newborns by Environmental Working Group

Website: www.ewg.org/research/body-burden-pollution-newborns
The purpose of the nonprofit Environmental Working Group is to empower people to live healthier lives in a healthier environment. This study shows how harmful industrial chemicals and pollutants reach babies during pregnancy through the umbilical cord.

Department of Energy—Whole House Ventilation

Website: https://www.energy.gov/energysaver/weatherize/
ventilation/whole-house-ventilation
This website offers descriptions and comparisons of whole-house ventilation systems that are designed to keep indoor air cleaner.

Harvard Health: Easy Ways You Can Improve Indoor Air Quality

Website: health.harvard.edu
When you reach the Harvard Health website, search for "indoor air quality." You will learn how to reduce indoor allergens that can trigger respiratory problems and other issues. Note that there is small monthly charge to access Harvard Health Online, which provides news from Harvard Medical School.

Health Impacts of Air Pollution

Website: www.edf.org/health/health-impacts-air-pollution
This article by the Environmental Defense Fund discusses the effects of environmental pollutants and how they contribute to a range of serious health disorders, from heart disease to diabetes to respiratory problems.

Lifehacker Best Air-Cleaning Plants

Website: https://lifehacker.com/this-graphic-shows-the-best-air
-cleaning-plants-accord-1705307836
This website provides information on common air contaminants and their sources and advises you of inexpensive household plants that will clean your indoor air according to the 1989 NASA Clean Air Study.

MedlinePlus Indoor Air Pollution

Website: https://medlineplus.gov/indoorairpollution.html
Provided by the National Library of Medicine, this article provides a summary of indoor air pollution sources and offers links to articles on improving air quality in your home and other important subjects.

Safe School Environmental Health Guidelines

Website: www.epa.gov/schools/read-state-school-environmental
-health-guidelines
The US Environmental Protection Agency (EPA) provides a wealth of information about environmental guidelines for schools and explains why these guidelines are so important.

Safer Choice Products

Website: https://www.epa.gov/saferchoice/products#sector=Home
Developed by the US Environmental Protection Agency, this website helps you find safe cleaning products and other products for use in your home or business.

Sherry Rogers. *Detoxify or Die.* DeWitt, NY: Prestige Publishing, 2002.

Written by Sherry F. Rogers, MD, an expert in environmental health, this book provides advice on coping with and eliminating toxins from the outside world.

■ LEAD

Lead Poisoning What Is It?

Website: health.harvard.edu
Access lead poisoning information by visiting the website, then entering "lead" in the search engine. This site provides the basics of what you need to know about lead poisoning: what it is as well as symptoms, diagnosis, treatment, and prevention.

Lead Poisoning Home Checklist

Website: www.epa.gov/sites/production/files/documents/
parent_checklist3.pdf
This site asks you specific questions to help you determine if your family is at risk for lead poisoning. If you find that you may be at risk, the site guides you to resources that can provide help.

■ MOLDS

Five Natural Home Remedies to Kill Mold

Website: https://emagazine.com/home-remedies-to-kill-mold/
This website from *E: The Environmental Magazine* shows how you can kill mold using five different natural remedies.

The Twelve Types of Mold

Website: https://aerindustries.com/blog/2017/03/28/
common-types-mold-in-home/
Visit this site to learn about twelve common types of mold that grow in homes. You'll read about the problems caused by mold and find photos that can help you identify the mold that is of concern to you.

■ VOLATILE ORGANIC COMPOUNDS (VOCS)

Volatile Organic Compounds' Impact on Indoor Air Quality

Website: www.epa.gov/indoor-air-quality-iaq/
volatile-organic-compounds-impact-indoor-air-quality
This website—provided by the EPA—offers important information you need to know about VOCs. You'll learn about the sources of VOCs, the health effects of these compounds, and most important, the steps you can take to reduce your exposure.

Volatile Organic Compounds in Your Home

Website: https://www.health.state.mn.us/communities/
environment/air/toxins/voc.htm
Hosted by the Minnesota Department of Health, this site provides easy-to-understand information about VOCs—what they are, where they're found, the effects they have on health, and how you can reduce your risk.

NUTRITION AND SUPPLEMENTS

Consumer.Lab.com

Website: www.consumerlab.com
Created by an organization that's independent of supplement manufacturers, ConsumerLab.com offers up-to-date research reports on various nutrients, including vitamins, minerals, and herbs. The website also compares many products by brand. An annual subscription fee is required for full access.

Eat a Rainbow

Website: https://www.roswellpark.org/cancertalk/201912/
health-benefits-phytochemicals-eat-rainbow
Provided by Roswell Park, the nation's first cancer center, Eat a Rainbow
lists the health benefits of the phytochemicals found in different foods.
Links allow you to explore other nutrition topics important to people
with cancer and to cancer survivors.

Environmental Working Group Shopper's Guide

Website: www.ewg.org
Visit the Environmental Working Group's website and click on the "Food"
icon. You'll learn about the produce that's most likely to be contaminated
with pesticides and find further information that can guide you in choosing safer foods for your family.

Harvard T.H. Chan of Public Health—The Nutrition Source

Website: www.hsph.harvard.edu/nutritionsource
This resource offers breaking nutrition news, articles on relevant subjects
such as sodium and fiber, tips for maintaining a healthy weight, and recipes that can be adapted for the American Heart Association Diet.

WebMD Food Calculator

Website: www.webmd.com/diet/healthtool-food-calorie-counter
This calculator quickly provides the calories, fat, carbohydrate, and protein contents for over 37,000 foods and beverages.

SPECIAL DIETS

■ AMERICAN HEART ASSOCIATION DIET

American Heart Association Diet and Lifestyle Recommendations

Website: www.heart.org
When you visit the website, perform a search for "American Heart
Association Diet and Lifestyle Recommendation." This resource pro-
vides specific guidelines for following the American Heart Association
Diet, and also offers information on the DASH Diet and Mediterranean
Diet.

■ DETOXIFICATION DIETS

Detox Diets: Cleansing the Body

Website: www.webmd.com

Go to WebMD and perform a search for "Detox Diets: Cleansing the Body by Jeanie Lerche Davis." The author discusses detox diets as a form of spring cleaning.

■ MEDITERRANEAN DIET

Healthline Mediterranean Diet Guide

Website: www.healthline.com

The Healthline website enables you to perform a search for "Mediterranean Diet 101: A Meal Plan and Beginner's Guide," which introduces you to the Mediterranean Diet and helps you choose healthy foods.

Mayo Clinic Mediterranean Diet

Website: www.mayoclinic.org

Once on the Mayo Clinic website, do a search for "Mediterranean Diet." Several pages will come up—even a Slide Show—so that you can choose what interests you. Suitable recipes for the diet are included.

■ DASH DIET

NIH DASH Eating Plan

Website: www.nhlbi.nih.gov/health-topics/dash-eating-plan

This website from the National Institutes of Health describes the benefits of the DASH eating plan and helps you get started.

Mayo Clinic DASH Diet

Website: www.mayoclinic.org

When you reach the Mayo Clinic website, search for the DASH Diet, and choose the topics that interest you. You'll find diet guidelines, sample menus, recipes, shopping tips, and more.

■ FASTING PROGRAMS

Healthline: 10 Evidence-Based Health Benefits of Intermittent Fasting

Website: https://www.healthline.com/nutrition/10-health-benefits-of-intermittent-fasting
Is intermittent fasting beneficial? This website explains the benefits that it offers.

Mayo Clinic Fasting

Website: www.mayoclinic.org
Enter "fasting" into the Mayo Clinic Search engine and many options will come up. Some of them are rather technical but others are more reader-friendly.

■ VEGETARIAN DIETS

Vegetarian Diet: How to Get the Best Nutrition

Website: www.mayoclinic.org
Enter "vegetarian diet plan" into the Mayo Clinic Search engine, and you will find guidelines, suggested daily amounts of each food group, and other information that will help you adopt a healthy vegetarian eating plan.

RECIPES

■ COOKBOOKS

American Heart Association. *The New American Heart Association Cookbook,* **ninth edition. Harmony, 2017.**
With 800 recipes, this is a great resource for anyone looking to improve cardiac health and lose weight.

America's Test Kitchen. *The Complete Mediterranean Cookbook.* **America's Test Kitchen, 2016.**
This comprehensive cookbook translates the famously healthy Mediterranean Diet for home cooks with a wide range of creative recipes that use easy-to-find ingredients.

Gaines, Fabiola Demps, and Roniece Weaver. *The New Soul Food: Cookbook for People with Diabetes,* second edition. **American Diabetes Association, 2006.**

The first African-American cookbook for people with diabetes, it offers more than 150 low-fat recipes, with each recipe including complete nutrition information so that you can determine if the dish would be suitable for you.

Jenkins-el, Nadira. *Vegan Soul Food Cookbook: Plant-Based No-Fuss Southern Favorites.* **Rockridge Press, 2020.**

In this cookbook, a vegan chef and holistic nutritionist offers plant-based recipes for a wide range of Southern favorites.

Moreno, Michelle. *The Dash Diet Cookbook.* **2020.**

A good cookbook for both new and experienced cooks, it offers 500 recipes for flavorful low-sodium meals.

O'Neill, Carolyn. *Southern Living Slim Down South Cookbook.* **TI Inc. Books, 2013.**

Written by a registered dietitian, this cookbook provides strategies, recipes, and expert tips for enjoying great Southern food while maintaining a healthier, balanced diet—without feeling deprived.

Taylor, Kathryne. *Love Real Food.* **Rodale Books, 2017.**

This cookbook offers more than 100 vegetarian favorites designed for everyone—vegetarians, vegans, and meat-eaters alike—with substitutions that will allow you to make meals special diet-friendly (gluten-free, dairy-free, and egg-free) whenever possible.

Willis, Virginia. *Lighten Up, Y'all: Classic Southern Recipes Made Healthy and Wholesome.* **Ten Speed Press, 2015.**

These recipes for Southern comfort foods are made lighter, healthier, and guilt-free, and yield delicious results.

■ RECIPE WEBSITES

Healthier Traditions Cookbooks

Website: www.transamericacenterforhealthstudies.com

This website allows you to download free Healthier Traditions Cookbooks, each of which features healthier twists on a different traditional cuisine, such as Italian, American, and soul foods.

Healthy Southern Recipes

Website: www.eatingwell.com/recipes/19701/cuisines-regions/usa/southern/
Hosted by Eating Well, this website includes healthier recipes for a wide range of dishes. Recipes, as well as guidelines and tips, are provided for a number of special eating plans and conditions, including the Mediterranean Diet, heart-healthy diets, and so on.

Soul Food Makeover—Heart Healthy African American Recipes

Website: https://www.nhlbi.nih.gov/health/educational/healthdisp/pdf/recipes/Recipes-African-American.pdf
A free website by the National Institutes of Health, it offers heart-healthy makeovers for traditional African-American foods.

DEVICES AND APPS

■ CONTINUOUS GLUCOSE MONITORING SYSTEMS

United States Medical Supply

Website: www.usmed.com/products/continuous-glucose-monitoring/
www.info.com/search
This website guides you to diabetes information and supplies, including information on continuous glucose monitoring systems such as DEXCOM and FreeStyle Libre.

■ STROKE ASSESSMENT APP

Stroke Riskometer

Website: www.strokeriskometer.com
Download this app, and you'll have an easy-to-use tool for assessing your risk of a stroke in the next five or ten years, as well as information on what you can do to reduce the risk. This app can also indicate your risk of heart attack, dementia, and diabetes.

References

Introduction

Bridges, KM. "Implicit bias and racial disparities in health care." *Human Rights Magazine*. Vol. 43, no. 3.

Ray, R. "Why are Blacks dying at higher rates from COVID-19?" Brookings Institute, 2020.

Chapter 1. The Gut-Microbiome-Brain Connection

Aggarwal, J, et al. "Probiotics and their effects on metabolic diseases: An update." *J Clin Diagn Res* (2013): Vol. 7, no. 1, 173–177.

Castro-Nallar, E, et al. "Composition, taxonomy and functional diversity of the oropharynx microbiome in individuals with schizophrenia and controls." *Peer Journal* (2015).

Cruickshank, et al. "Sick genes, sick individuals or sick populations with chronic disease? The emergence of diabetes and high blood pressure in African-origin populations." *International Journal of Epidemiology* (2001): Vol. 30, no.1, 111–117.

David, LA, et al. "Diet rapidly and reproducibly alters the human gut microbiome." *Nature* (2014): Vol. 505, 559–563.

De Filippo, C, et al. "Impact of diet in shaping gut microbiota revealed by a comparative study in children from Europe and rural Africa." *Proc Natl Acad Sci* (2010): Vol. 107, 14691–6.

De Gottardi, A, McCoy, KD. "Evaluation of the gut barrier to intestinal bacteria in non-alcoholic fatty liver disease." *J Hepatol* (2011): Vol. 55, 1181–1183.

Gorbach, SL. "Microbiology of the Gastrointestinal Tract." In *Medical Microbiology*, fourth edition. Galveston: University of Texas Medical Branch at Galveston, 1996.

Gunnars, K. "20 Foods That Are Bad for Your Health." 2019. https://www.healthline.com/nutrition/20-foods-to-avoid-like-the-plague

Iversen, S, et al. *Principles of Neural Science*. New York: Mc-Graw Hill, 2000.

Klok, MD, et al. "The role of leptin and ghrelin in the regulation of food intake and body weight in humans: A review." *Obes Rev* (2007): Vol. 8, 21–34.

Krack, A, et al. "The importance of the gastrointestinal system in the pathogenesis of heart failure." *Eur Heart J* (2005): Vol. 26, 2368–2374.

Lam, V, et al. "Intestinal microbiota determine severity of myocardial infarction in rats." *FASEB J* (2012): 1727–35.

Ley, RE, et al. "Microbial ecology: Human gut microbes associated with obesity." *Nature* (2006): Vol. 444, 1022–1023.

Naseribafrouei, A, Hestad, K, Avershina, E, Sekelja, M, et al. "Correlation between the human fecal microbiota and depression." *Neurogastroenterol Motil* (2014): Vol. 26, no. 8, 1155–62.

Petra, AI, et al. "Gut-microbiota-brain axis and its effect in neuropsychiatric disorders with suspected immune dysregulation." *Clin Ther* (2015): Vol. 3, no. 7, 984–95.

Schmidt, A, et al. *Human Physiology*, second edition. New York: Springer-Verlag, 1989, 333–370.

Sevelsted, A, et al. "Cesarean section and chronic immune disorders." *Pediatrics* (2015): Vol. 135, no.1, e92–8.

Sharon, G, et al. "The central nervous system and the gut microbiome." *Cell* (2016): Vol. 167, no. 4, 915–32.

Singh, RK, et al. "Influence of diet on the gut microbiome and implications for human health." *J Trans Med* (2017): Vol. 15, 73.

Ulrich-Lai, YM, et al. "Sympatho-adrenal activity and hypothalamic-pituitary-adrenal axis regulation." In Steckler, T, Kalin, NH, Reul, J, (ed.). *Handbook of Stress and the Brain*. Amsterdam: Elsevier B.V., 2005, 419–435.

Weir, TL, et al. "Stool microbiome and metabolome differences between colorectal cancer patients and healthy adults." *PLoS ONE* (2013): Vol. 8, e70803.

Wu, HJ, Wu, E. "The role of gut microbiota in immune homeostasis and autoimmunity." *Gut Microbes* (2012): Vol. 3, no. 1, 4–14.

Zhang, YJ, et al."Impacts of gut bacteria on human health and diseases." *Int J Mol Sci.* (2015): Vol. 16, no. 4, 7493–7519.

Chapter 2. Obesity

Agarwal, N, et al. "Toxic exposure in America: Estimating fetal and infant health outcomes from 14 years of TRI reporting." *Journal of Health Economics* (2010): Vol. 29, 557–574.

Ahima, RS, et al. "Leptin." *Annu Rev Physiol* (2000): Vol. 62, 413–437.

Bell, M, Ebisu, K. "Environmental inequality in exposures to airborne particulate matter components in the United States." *Environmental Health Perspectives* (2012): Vol. 120, no. 12, 1699–1704.

Centers for Disease Control and Prevention. "Health of Black or African American non-Hispanic population." National Center for Health Statistics (2019).

Centers for Disease Control and Prevention. Office of Minority Health. "Infant mortality statistics from the 2017 period linked birth/infant death data set." *National Vital Statistics Reports* (2019): Table 5.

Centers for Disease Control and Prevention. Office of Minority Health. "Infant mortality statistics from the 2017 period linked birth/infant death data set." *National Vital Statistics Reports* (2019): Table 2.

Cluny, NL, et al. "Cannabinoid signalling regulates inflammation and energy balance: The importance of the brain-gut axis." *Brain Behav Immu* (2012): Vol. 26, 691–698.

Cooper, JA, et al. "Serum leptin levels in obese males during over-and under-feeding." *Obesity* (2009): Vol. 17, 2149–2154.

De los Reyes-Gavilan, CG, et al. "Development of functional foods to fight against obesity: Opportunities for probiotics and prebiotics." *Agro Food Ind Hi Tech* (2014): Vol. 25, 35–39.

"Ethnicity and Health in America Series. Obesity in the African-American Community." American Psychological Association.

Goldstein, BJ, Scalia, R. "Adiponectin: A novel adipokine linking adipocytes and vascular function." *J Clin Endocrinol Metab* (2004): Vol. 89, 2563–2568.

Gupte, M, et al. "Angiotensin converting enzyme 2 contributes to sex differences in the development of obesity hypertension in C57BL/6 mice." *Arterioscler Thromb Vasc Biol* (2012): Vol. 3, 1392–1399.

Hildebrandt, MA, et al. "High-fat diet determines the composition of the murine gut microbiome independently of obesity." *Gastroenterology* (2009): Vol. 137, 1716–24.

"How obesity has become a part of black culture." *The Grio* (2020).

Jackson, E, et al. "Adipose tissue as a site of toxin accumulation." *Compr Physiol* (2017): Vol. 7, no. 4, 1085–1135.

Johnston, CS, et al. "Vitamin C elevates red blood cell glutathione in healthy adults." *Am J Clin Nutr* (1993): Vol. 58, no. 1, 103–5.

Kantartzis, K, et al. "The association between plasma adiponectin and insulin sensitivity in humans depends on obesity." *Obes Res* (2005): Vol. 13, 1683–1691.

Karlsson, C, et al. "Human adipose tissue expresses angiotensinogen and enzymes required for its conversion to angiotensin II." *J Clin Endocrinol Metab* (1998): Vol. 83, 3925–3929.

Kelishadi, R, et al. "A randomized triple-masked controlled trial on the effects of synbiotics on inflammation markers in overweight children." *J Pediatr* (2014): Vol. 90, 161–168.

Kirby, RS. "The US Black-White infant mortality gap: Marker of deep inequities." *Am J Public Health* (2017): Vol. 107, no. 5, 644–645.

Lanphear, BP, et al. "Protecting children from environmental toxins." *PLoS Medicine* (2005): Vol. 3, no. 1, 203–208.

Latini, G, et al. "Toxic environment and obesity pandemia: Is there a relationship?" *Ital J Pediatr* (2010): Vol. 36, no. 8.

Lieber, CS, Packer, L. "S-Adenolsylmethionine: Molecular, biological, and clinical aspects—an introduction." *Am J Clin Nutr* (2002): Vol. 76, no. 5, 1148S–50S.

Mozaffarian, D, et al. "Changes in diet and lifestyle and long-term weight gain in women and men." *N Engl J Med* (2011): Vol. 364, 2392–2404.

Pendyala, L, Creaven, PJ. "Pharmacokinetic and pharmacodynamic studies of N-acetylcysteine, a potential chemopreventive agent during a phase I trial." *Cancer Epidemiol Biomarkers Prev* (1995): Vol. 4, no. 3, 245–51.

Pizzorno, J. "Glutathione!" *Integr Med* (2014): Vol. 13, no. 1, 8–12.

Pohl, HR, et al. "Health effects classification and its role in the derivation of minimal risk levels: Developmental effects." *Regulatory Toxicology and Pharmacology* (1998): Vol. 28, no. 1, 55–60.

Woodruff, TJ, et al. "Environmental chemicals in pregnant women in the United States. NHANES 2003–2004." *Environmental Health Perspectives* (2011): Vol. 119, no. 6, 878–885.

Chapter 3. Hypertension

Forde, AT, et al. "Discrimination and hypertension risk among African Americans in the Jackson Heart Study." *Hypertension* (2020): Vol. 76, 715–723.

Harvard Men's Health Watch. Reading the new blood pressure guidelines. Updated: June 1, 2020. Published: April, 2018. https://www.health.harvard.edu/heart-health/reading-the-new-blood-pressure-guidelines

Liu, T. "High blood pressure linked to short-, long-term exposure to some air pollutants." *Science News* (2016).

Luyckx, VA, Brenner, BM. "Birth weight, malnutrition and kidney-associated outcomes—a global concern." *Nat Rev Nephrol.* Vol. 11, no. 3, 135–49.

NIH. "Gene variants linked to blood pressure in African Americans." *NIH Research Matters* (2009).

Sanders, AP, et al. "Perinatal and childhood exposure to environmental chemicals and blood pressure in children: A review of literature." *Pediatr Res* (2018): Vol. 84, no. 2, 165–180.

Tello, M. "New high blood pressure guidelines: Think your blood pressure is fine? Think again. . ." Harvard Health Blog (2019).

Zilbermint, M, et al. "Genetics of hypertension in African Americans and others of African descent." *Int J Mol Sci* (2019): Vol. 20, no. 5, 1081.

Chapter 4. Diabetes

Alemzadeh, R, et al. "Hypovitaminosis D in obese children and adolescents: Relationship with adiposity, insulin sensitivity, ethnicity, and season." *Metabolism* (2008): Vol. 57, no. 2, 183–191.

Alfonso, B, et al. "Vitamin D in diabetes mellitus–A new field of knowledge poised for D-velopment." *Diabetes Metab Res Rev* (2009): Vol. 25, no. 5, 417–419.

Al-Thakafy, HS, et al. "Alterations of erythrocyte free radical defense system, heart tissue lipid peroxidation, and lipid concentration in streptozotocininduced diabetic rats under coenzyme Q_{10} supplementation." *Saudi Med J* (2004): Vol. 25, no. 12, 1824–1830.

Anderson, RA, Preuss, HG. "Chromium update: Examining recent literature 1997–1998." *Current Opinion in Clinical Nutrition and Metabolic Care* (1998): Vol. 1, no. 6, 509–512.

Anderson, RA, et al. "Isolation and characterization of polyphenol type-a polymers from cinnamon with insulin-like biological activity." *J Agri Food Chem* (2004): Vol. 52, no. 1, 65–70.

Boudou, P, et al. "Hyperglycaemia acutely decreases circulating dehydroepiandrosterone levels in healthy men." *Clinical Endocrinology* (2006): Vol. 64, no. 1, 46–52.

Chandalia, M, et al. "Beneficial effects of high dietary fiber intake in patients with Type 2 diabetes mellitus." *New England Journal of Medicine* (2000): Vol. 342, 1392–1398.

Crespy, V, Williamson, GA. "Review of the health effects of green tea catechins in in vivo animal models." *J Nutr* (2004): Vol. 134, 3431S–3440S.

Csiszar, A, and Ungvari, Z. "Endothelial dysfunction and vascular inflammation in Type 2 diabetes: Interaction of AGE/RAGE and TNF signaling." *Am J Physiol Heart Circ Physiol* (2008): Vol. 295, no. 2, H475–H476.

Ghosh, D, et al. "Role of chromium supplementation in Indians with Type 2 diabetes mellitus." *The Journal of Nutritional Biochemistry* (2002): Vol. 13, no. 11, 690–697.

Guideri, F, et al. "Effects of acetyl-l-carnitine on cardiac dysautonomia in Rett syndrome: Prevention of sudden death?" *Pediatric Cardiology* (2005): Vol. 26, no. 5, 574–577.

Henriksen, EJ, et al. "Stimulation by alpha-lipoic acid of glucose transport activity in skeletal muscle of lean and obese zucker rats." *Life Sciences* (1997): Vol. 61, no. 8, 805–812.

Hodgson, JM, Watts, GF. "Can coenzyme Q_{10} improve vascular function and blood pressure? Potential for effective therapeutic reduction in vascular oxidative stress." *BioFactors* (2003): Vol. 18, no. 1–4, 129–136.

Imparl-Radosevich, J, et al. "Regulation of PTP-1 and insulin receptor kinase by fractions from cinnamon: Implications for cinnamon regulation of insulin signaling." *Horm Res* (1998): Vol. 50, no. 3, 177–182.

Jones, RD, et al. "Testosterone and atherosclerosis in aging men: Purported association and clinical implications." *American Journal of Cardiovascular Drugs* (2005): Vol. 56, no. 3, 141–154.

Laditka, SB, et al. "Health care use of individuals with diabetes in an employer-based insurance population." *Arch Intern Med* (2001): Vol. 161, no. 10, 1301–1308.

Lee, J. H, et al. "Vitamin D deficiency an important, common, and easily treatable cardiovascular risk factor?" *J Am Coll Cardiol* (2008): Vol. 52, no. 24, 1949–1956.

Littorin, B, et al. "Lower levels of plasma 25-hydroxyvitamin D among young adults at diagnosis of autoimmune Type 1 diabetes compared with control subjects: Results from the nationwide Diabetes Incidence Study in Sweden (DISS)." *Diabetologia* (2006): Vol. 49, no. 12, 2847–2852.

Medina, MC, et al. "Dehydroepiandrosterone increases beta-cell mass and improves the glucose-induced insulin secretion by pancreatic islets from aged rats." *FEBS Lett* (2006): Vol. 580, no. 1, 285–290.

Mingrone, G. "Carnitine in Type 2 diabetes." *Annals of the New York Academy of Sciences* (2004): Vol. 1033, 99–107.

Murase, T, et al. "Green tea extract improves endurance capacity and increases muscle lipid oxidation in mice." *Am J Physiol Regul Integr Comp Physiol* (2005): Vol. 288, R708–R715.

Nurulain, TZ. "Green tea and its polyphenolic catechins: Medicinal uses in cancer and noncancer applications." *Life Sciences* (2006): Vol. 78, no. 18, 2073–2080.

Okuda, T, et al. "Inhibitory effect of tannins on direct-acting mutation." *Chem Pharm Bull* (1984): Vol. 32, 3755–3758.

Penckofer, S, et al. "Vitamin D and diabetes: Let the sunshine in." *Diabetes Educ* (2008): Vol. 34, no. 6, 939–944.

Watts, GF, et al. "Coenzyme Q_{10} improves endothelial dysfunction of the brachial artery in Type II diabetes mellitus." *Diabetologia* (2002): Vol. 45, no. 3, 420–426.

Wright, E, et al. "Oxidative stress in Type 2 diabetes: The role of fasting and postprandial gylcemia." *Int J Clin Pract* (2006): Vol. 60, no. 3, 308–314.

Yamashita, R, et al. "Effects of dehydroepiandrosterone on gluconeogenic enzymes and glucose uptake in human hepatoma cell line, HepG2." *Endocr J* (2005): Vol. 52, no. 6, 727–753.

Zittermann, A, et al. "Circulating calcitriol concentrations and total mortality." *Clin Chem* (2009): Vol. 55, no. 6, 1163–1170.

Chapter 5. Cardiovascular Disease

Aroor, S, et al." BE-FAST (balance, eyes, face, arm, speech, time): Reducing the proportion of strokes missed using the FAST mnemonic." *Stroke* (2017): Vol. 48, no. 2, 479–481.

Haglund, O, et al. "The effects of fish oil on triglycerides, cholesterol, fibrinogen and malondialdehyde in humans supplemented with vitamin E." *J Nutr* (1991): Vol. 21, no. 2, 165–9.

Lefebvre, KM, et al. "Disparities in amputations in minorities." *Clinical Orthopaedics and Related Research* (2011): Vol. 469, 1941–1950.

Parmar, P, et al. "The Stroke Riskometer app: Validation of a data collection tool and stroke risk predictor." *Int J Stroke* (2015): Vol. 10, no. 2, 231–244.

Chapter 6. Kidney Disease

Ebele, M, et al. "You are just now telling us about this? African American perspectives of testing for genetic susceptibility to kidney disease." *JASN* (2019): Vol. 30, no. 4, 526–530.

Haglund, O, et al. "The effects of fish oil on triglycerides, cholesterol, fibrinogen and malondialdehyde in humans supplemented with vitamin E." *J Nutr* (1991): Vol. 21, no. 2, 165–9.

Chapter 7. Cancer

American Cancer Society. "Cancer Facts and Figures for African Americans." 2019–2021.

Barbany, G, et al. "Cell-free tumour DNA testing for early detection of cancer–A potential future tool." *J Intern Med* (2019): Vol. 286, no. 2, 118–136.

Dess, R, et al. "Association of Black race with prostate cancer: Specific and other-cause mortality." *JAMA Oncol* (2019): Vol. 5, no. 7, 975–983.

Dufault, Renee Joy. *Unsafe at Any Meal*. Garden City Park, NY: Square One Publishers, Inc., 2017.

Feldman, D, et al. *Dietary Reference Intakes for Calcium and Vitamin D*. Washington, DC: National Academies Press, 2011.

Feldman D, et al. "The role of vitamin D in reducing cancer risk and progression." *Nat Rev Cancer* (2014): Vol. 14, no. 5, 342–57.

Fiala, C, et al. "New approaches for detecting cancer with circulating cell-free DNA." *BMC Med* (2019): Vol. 17, no.1, 159.

Giovannucci, E, et al. "Calcium and fructose intake in relation to risk of prostate cancer." *Cancer Res* (1998): Vol. 58, no. 3, 442–7.

Grant, WB, "Review of recent advances in understanding the role of vitamin D in reducing cancer risk: Breast, colorectal, prostate, and overall cancer." *Anticancer Res* (2020): Vol. 40, no. 1, 491–499.

Gu, D, et al. "A comprehensive approach to the profiling of the cooked meat carcinogens 2-amino-3,8-dimethylimidazo[4,5-f]quinoxaline, 2-amino-1-methyl-6-phenylimidazo[4,5-b]pyridine, and their metabolites in human urine." *Chem Res Toxicol* (2010): Vol. 3, no. 4, 788–801.

Huss, L, et al. "Vitamin D receptor expression in invasive breast tumors and breast cancer survival." *Breast Cancer Research* (2019): Vol. 21.

International Agency for Research on Cancer. "Red meat and processed meat monographs on the evaluation of carcinogenic risks to humans." *IARC* (2018): Vol. 114.

John, EM, et al. "Meat consumption, cooking practices, meat mutagens, and risk of prostate cancer." *Nutr Cancer* (2011): Vol. 63, 525–537.

Manson, JE, et al. "Vitamin D supplements and prevention of cancer and cardiovascular disease." *NEJM* (2019): Vol. 380, 33–44.

Martin, R. *Vitamin D and Prostate Cancer.* World Cancer Research Fund International, 2017.

McDermott, A. "Can vitamin D deficiency lead to prostate cancer?" *Healthline Review* (2017).

Punnen, S, et al." Impact of meat consumption, preparation, and mutagens on aggressive prostate cancer." *PLoS One* (2011): Vol. 6, e27711.

Ross, AC, et al. "Dietary reference intakes for calcium and vitamin D. what clinicians need to know." Journal of Clinical Endocrinology & Metabolism (2011): Vol. 96, no. 1, 53–58.

Rowland, GW, et al. "Calcium intake and prostate cancer among African Americans: Effect modification by vitamin D receptor calcium absorption genotype." *J Bone Miner Res* (2012): Vol. 27, no. 1, 187–94.

Schuurman, AG, et al. "Animal products, calcium and protein and prostate cancer risk in The Netherlands Cohort Study." *Br J Cancer* (1998): Vol. 80, 1107–1113.

Shapses, SA, et al. "The effect of obesity on the relationship between serum parathyroid hormone and 25-hydroxyvitamin D in women." *J Clin Endocrinol Metab* (2013): Vol. 98, E886–E890.

Sinha, R, et al. "Heterocyclic amine content in beef cooked by different methods to varying degrees of doneness and gravy made from meat drippings." *Food Chem Toxicol (1998):* Vol. 36, no. 4, 279–87.

Wambui, G, et al. "Dietary factors and risk of advanced prostate cancer." *Eur J Cancer Prev* (2014): Vol. 23, no. 2, 96–109.

Chapter 8. The Aging Process

Castillo, M. E, et al. "Effect of calcifediol treatment and best available therapy versus best available therapy on intensive care unit admission and mortality among patients hospitalized for COVID-19: A pilot randomized clinical study." *J Steroid Biochem and Mol Biol* (2020): Vol. 203.

"Vitamin D protects cells from stress that can lead to cancer." *International Journal of Cancer* (2008).

Chapter 9. Nutrition and Diets

Booth, J. "These Foods Have Been Banned in Other Countries, But Are Still Legal in the United States." 2019. https://soyummy.com/banned-foods/

Chapter 10. Environmental Health

Agency for Toxic Substances and Disease Registry. "Lead Toxicity. Where Is Lead Found?" (2021).

Agency for Toxic Substances and Disease Registry. "Toxicity. What Is the Biological Fate of Lead in the Body?" (2019).

American Chemistry Council. "Lifecycle of a plastic product." https://plastics.americanchemistry.com/Lifecycle-of-a-Plastic-Product/

Anton, SD, et al. "Flipping the metabolic switch: Understanding and applying the health benefits of fasting." *Obesity* (2018): Vol. 26, 254–268.

Asthma and Allergy Foundation of America. "Asthma Disparities in America." (2020).

Asthma and Allergy Foundation of America. "Ethnic Disparities in the Burden and Treatment of Asthma." (2005).

Bailey, DG, et al. "Grapefruit juice—Drug interactions." *Br J Clin Pharmacol* (1998): Vol. 46, no. 2, 101–110.

Baynes, RE, Riviere, JE. "Distribution and Pharmacokinetics Models." In *Pesticide Biotransformation and Disposition*. Academic Press, 2012.

Bornehag, CG, et al. "Dampness in buildings and health. Dampness at home as a risk factor for symptoms among 10,851 Swedish children. (DBH-STEP 1)." *Indoor Air* (2005): Vol. 15, Suppl. 10, 48–55.

Canfield, RL, et al. "Intellectual impairment in children with blood lead concentrations below 10 μg per deciliter." *N Engl J Med* (2003): Vol. 348, 1517–1526.

Cappuccio, FP, et al. "Sleep duration and all-cause mortality: A systematic review and meta-analysis of prospective studies." *Sleep* (2010): Vol. 33, no. 5, 585–592.

Centers for Disease Control and Prevention. "Biomonitoring. Phthalates Factsheet."

Centers for Disease Control and Prevention. "Life Expectancy."

Chronic Hazard Advisory Panel On Phthalates and Phthalate Alternatives. "Report to the U.S. Consumer Product Safety Commission." July, 2014.

de Cabo, R, Mattson, M P. "Effects of intermittent fasting on health, aging, and disease." *N Engl J Med* (2019): Vol. 381, 2541–2551.

EESI. "Fact Sheet—A Brief History of Octane in Gasoline: From Lead to Ethanol." (2016).

Environmental Protection Agency. "Lead Regulations."

Environmental Protection Agency. "Particulate Matter (PM) Basics."

Environmental Working Group. "Body Burden: The Pollution in Newborns." (2005).

Food and Drug Administration. "Grapefruit Juice and Some Drugs Don't Mix."

Grineski, SE, Collins, TW. "Geographic and social disparities in exposure to air neurotoxicants at U.S. public schools." *Environ Res* (2018): Vol. 161, 580–587.

Guern, CL. "When the Mermaids Cry: The Great Plastic Tide." (2019).

Harvie, M, et al. "The effect of intermittent energy and carbohydrate restriction v. daily energy restriction on weight loss and metabolic disease risk markers in overweight women." *Br J Nutr* (2013): Vol. 110, 1534–1547.

Jaakkola, JJK, et al. "Interior surface materials and asthma in adults: A population-based incident case-control study." *American Journal of Epidemiology* (2006): Vol. 164, no.8, 742–749.

Kolarik, B, et al. "The association between phthalates in dust and allergic diseases among Bulgarian children." *Environmental Health Perspectives* (2008): Vol. 116, no. 1, 98–103.

Larsson, M, et al. "Associations between indoor environmental factors and parental-reported autistic spectrum disorders in children 6-8 years of age." *Neurotoxicology* (2009): Vol. 30, no. 5, 822–31.

Mattson, MP, et al. "Intermittent metabolic switching, neuroplasticity and brain health." *Nat Rev Neurosci* (2018): Vol. 19, 63–80.

Mattson, MP, Arumugam, TV. "Hallmarks of brain aging: Adaptive and pathological modification by metabolic states." *Cell Metab* (2018): Vol. 27, 1176–1199.

Mayo Clinic. "Lead Poisoning."

Mitchell, JN. "Black male, female life expectancy lowest across the city." *Tribune* (2020).

Needleman, HL. "History of Lead Poisoning in the World." CDC: (1999).

Newkirk,VR. "Trump's EPA concludes environmental racism is real." *The Atlantic* (2018).

Norbäck, D, et al. "Asthma symptoms in relation to measured building dampness in upper concrete floor construction, and 2-ethyl-1-hexanol in indoor air." *International Journal of Tuberculosis and Lung Disease* (2000): Vol. 4, No. 11, 1016–1025.

O'Connell, K. "Effects of insomnia on the body." *Healthline* (2018).

Office of Disease Prevention and Health Promotion. "Healthy People."

Passarelli, GR. World Health Organization. "Sick building syndrome: An overview to raise awareness." *Journal of Building Appraisal* (2009): Vol. 5, 55–66.

Pelleyu, J. "Number of chemicals in commerce has been vastly underestimated." *C&EN* (2020): Vol. 98, no. 7

National Research Council. "Phthalates and Cumulative Risk Assessment: The Tasks Ahead." (2008).

Pinola, M. "This graphic shows the best air-cleaning plants, according to

NASA." https://lifehacker.com/this-graphic-shows-the-best-air-cleaning-plants-accord-1705307836

Raman, R. "Can You Microwave Styrofoam, and Should You?" (2020).

Schroder, AP, et al. "Lead toxicity and chelation therapy." *US Pharm* (2015): Vol. 40, no. 5, 40–44.

Shu, H, et al. "PVC-flooring at home and development of asthma among young children in Sweden, a 10-year follow-up." *Indoor Air* (2013): Vol. 24, no. 3.

Spiegel, K, et al. "Sleep curtailment in healthy young men is associated with decreased leptin levels, elevated ghrelin levels, and increased hunger and appetite." *Ann Intern Med* (2004): Vol. 141, 846–50.

Spiegel, K, et al. "Sleep loss: A novel risk factor for insulin resistance and Type 2 diabetes." *J Appl Physiol* (2005): Vol. 99, 2008–19.

Spiegel, K, et al. "The metabolic consequences of sleep deprivation." *Sleep Med Rev* (2007): Vol. 11, 163–78.

Taheri, S, et al. "Short sleep duration is associated with reduced leptin, elevated ghrelin, and increased body mass index." *PLoS Med* (2004) Vol. 1, e62.

Tessum, CW, et al. "Inequity in consumption of goods and services adds to racial-ethnic disparities in air pollution exposure." *PNAS* (2019): Vol. 116, no. 13, 6001–6006.

Tuomainen, A, et al. "Indoor air quality and health problems associated with damp floor coverings in an office building." *International Archives of Occupational and Environmental Health* (2004): Vol. 77, no. 3, 222–226.

Wang, Z, et al. "Toward a global understanding of chemical pollution: A first comprehensive analysis of national and regional chemical inventories." *Environ Sci Technol* (2020): Vol. 54, 2575–2584.

WHO. "Dioxins and Their Effects on Human Health."

Whyatt, RM, et al. "Asthma in inner-city children at 5–11 years of age and prenatal exposure to phthalates: The Columbia Center for Children's Environmental Health Cohort." *Environ Health Perspect* (2014): Vol. 122, 1141–1146.

Wolf, L, Wolf, T. "Music and health care: A paper commissioned by the Musical Connections Program of Carnegie Hall's Weill Music Institute." (2011).

Chapter 11. Sickle Cell Disease

Brown, B, et al. "The association between vitamin D deficiency and hospitalization outcomes in pediatric patients with sickle cell disease." *Blood Cells Mol Dis* (2020): Vol. 82.

Centers for Disease Control and Prevention. "Complications and Treatments of Sickle Cell Disease."

Centers for Disease Control and Prevention. "Disparities in Oral Health." (2020).

Cleveland Clinic. "Sickle Cell Disease: Outlook/Prognosis."

Daak, AA, et al. "Effect of omega-3 (n-3) fatty acid supplementation in patients with sickle cell anemia: Randomized, double-blind, placebo-controlled trial." *Am J Clin Nutr* (2013): Vol. 97, no. 1, 37–44.

GBD. "Global, regional, and national incidence, prevalence, and years lived with disability for 310 diseases and injuries, 1990–2015: A systematic analysis for the Global Burden of Disease Study." *Lancet* (2015): Vol. 388, no. 10053, 1545–1602.

Herrick, JB. "Peculiar elongated and sickle-shaped red blood corpuscles in a case of severe anemia." *Yale J Biol Med.* (1910): Vol. 74, no. 3, 179–84.

Hoffman, KM, et al. "Racial bias in pain assessment and treatment recommendations, and false beliefs about biological differences between blacks and whites." *Proc Natl Acad Sci of the USA* (2016): Vol. 113, no.16, 4296–4301.

MedicineNet. "Hemoglobin vs. Hematocrit." (2020).

National Heart, Lung and Blood Institute. "Sickle Cell Patient's Recovery After Gene Therapy Heightens Hopes for a Cure."(2019).

National Heart, Lung and Blood Institute. "Opioid Crisis Adds to Pain of Sickle Cell Patients." (2017).

National Institutes of Health. "Backgrounder: NIH Collaboration on Gene-Based Cures for SCD and HIV."

Pray, LA. "Discovery of DNA structure and function: Watson and Crick." *Nature Education* (2008).

Rees, DC, et al. "Sickle-cell disease." *Lancet* (2010): Vol. 376, no. 9757, 2018–31.

Serjeant, GR. "One hundred years of sickle cell disease." *British Journal of Haematology* (2010): Vol. 151, no. 5, 425–9.

Starling, S. "The levee breaks—Initial reports of AIDS." *Milestones* (2018).

Starr, Douglas. *Blood: An Epic History of Medicine and Commerce.* New York: Harper Perennial, 2000.

Thom, CS, et al. "Hemoglobin variants: Biochemical properties and clinical correlates." *Cold Spring Harb Perspect Med* (2013): Vol. 3, no. 3. (3) a011858.

Tisdale, JF, et al. "Treating sickle cell anemia." *Science* (2020): Vol. 367, no. 6483, 1198–1199.

Winter, WP. "A Brief History of Sickle Cell Disease."

Chapter 12. Oral Health

Assari, S, Hani, N. "Household income and children's unmet dental care need: Blacks' diminished return." *Dentistry Journal* (2018): Vol. 6, no. 217.

Bissett, G. "Black Lives Matter—Experiences from the dental profession." *Dentistry* (2020).

Centers for Disease Control and Prevention. "What Dental Professionals Would Like Team Members to Know About Oral Health and Diabetes." (2020).

Duhaime-Ross, A. "Black kids in the US have twice as many untreated cavities as white ones." (2015).

Dunbar, S. "Oral Care Training for Older Adults." (2020).

Feinberg, M. "Minority oral health in America: Despite progress, disparities persist." American Dental Association.

Fernandes, J, et al. "Periodontal disease status in Gullah African Americans with Type 2 diabetes living in South Carolina." *Journal of Periodontology.* (2020).

Luo, H, et al. "Forty-year trends in tooth loss among American adults with and without diabetes mellitus: An age-period-cohort analysis." *Prev Chronic Dis* (2015): Vol. 12.

"Racial Disparity in Dental Care. The Numbers Tell the Story." *Group Dentistry Now* (2020).

Rawson, K. "10 Daily tips to improve overall oral health." *Health Prep* (2016).

Sabbah, W, et al. "Racial discrimination and uptake of dental services among American adults." *International Journal of Environmental Research and Public Health* (2019): Vol. 16, no. 9, 1558.

Sohn, H. "Racial and ethnic disparities in health insurance coverage: Dynamics of gaining and losing coverage over the life-course." *Population Research and Policy Review* (2017): Vol. 36, no. 2, 181–201.

Stetler, C. "Rare Gum Disease Among African-American Children is Focus of Rutgers Study." *Rutgers Today.* (2015).

Conclusion

"African Americans Law and Legal Definitions." USLegal.com.

Baharian, S, et al. "The Great Migration and African-American genomic diversity." *PLOS Genetics.* (2016).

Campbell, MC, Tishkoff, SA. "African genetic diversity: Implications for human demographic history, modern human origins, and complex disease mapping." *Annu Rev Genomics Hum Genet* (2008): Vol. 9, 403–433.

Census Bureau. "The Black Population." (2010).

Conroy, M, Bacon, P. "There's a huge gap in how Republicans and Democrats see discrimination." FiveThirtyEight Blog (2020).

FitzGerald, C, Hurst, S. "Implicit bias in healthcare professionals: A systematic review." *BMC Medical Ethics* (2017).

Forde, AT, et al. "Discrimination and hypertension risk among African Americans in the Jackson Heart Study." *Hypertension* (2020): Vol. 76, 715–723.

Greenwood, BN, Hardeman, RR. "Physician–patient racial concordance and disparities in birthing mortality for newborns." *PNAS* (2020): Vol. 117, no. 35.

Griffith, DM, et al. "Ethnicity, nativity and the health of American Blacks." *J Health Care Poor Underserved* (2011).

Salvaggio, JE. *New Orleans' Charity Hospital: A Story of Physicians, Politics, and Poverty.* Baton Rouge, LA: LSU Press, 1992.

"Slave Health on Plantations in the United States." Wikipedia.

Smedley, BD. "Unequal treatment: Confronting racial and ethnic disparities in health care." *IOM* (2003): Appendix D.

Tello, M. "Racism and discrimination in health care: Providers and patients." Harvard Health Blog (2020).

Williams, DR, Rucker, TD. "Understanding and addressing racial disparities in health care." *Health Care Financ Rev* (2000): Vol. 21, no. 4, 75–90.

Winful, T. "Reconstructing Africa's Evolutionary Histories: DNA Collection, Coding, Analysis, and Interpretation." University of North Carolina at Charlotte (2018).

BLACK HEALTH TIMELINES

From Africa to the Pre-Civil War Years

Owens, DC. "Medical Bondage: Race, Gender, and the Origins of American Gynecology." University of Georgia Press, 2017.

The Great Migration

Black, DA, et al. "The impact of the great migration on mortality of African Americans: Evidence from the deep south." *American Economic Review* (2015): Vol. 105, no. 2, 477–503.

Byrd, WM, Clayton, LA. "An American health dilemma: A history of Blacks in the health system." *Journal of the National Medical Association* (1992): Vol. 84, No. 2, 108.

The Red Cross

Pilgrim, D. "The Truth About the Death of Charles Drew." Ferris State University, 2004.

About the Author

Richard W. Walker, Jr., MD, was born in New York City and raised in the Johnson Projects of Spanish Harlem. As a child, he suffered from many different medical conditions, including pneumonia, appendicitis, heart murmurs, and more. From his frequent visits to his "favorite" hospital, Columbia Presbyterian in Washington Heights, he still recalls the image of black stethoscopes against all-white uniforms. It was through these experiences that his desire to become a physician was born.

By the time he was in high school, however, his goal was simply to graduate. His tough neighborhood, the discouragement of school counselors, and an undiagnosed case of dyslexia all made him see himself as "not college material," despite his notably high I.Q. After barely squeaking by, he received his high school diploma only to drop out of community college due to poor grades. Seeking direction, he chose to join the Armed Forces. It was during this time that he met the person who would change his life, his future wife, Marvia. The two were married after dating for only three months.

Thanks to his success as a member of the United States Air Force, and Marvia's persistence and inspiration, he decided to give college another try. He began taking courses one at a time and performed very well in all of them. By the time he was honorably discharged from the Air Force, he had a full semester's credits behind him. In 1969, he enrolled at John Jay College of Criminal Justice in New York City, graduating with a bachelor's degree in forensic science in 1971, all while working a full-time job and supporting a family of four. While studying for a master's degree at the same institution, he was approached by Professor Alexander Joseph, PhD, the dean of the science department, who had learned of the training the promising student had received as a combat medic in the Armed Forces. Recognizing his potential, Dr. Joseph strongly encouraged him to go to medical school. With very little money and lots of bills to pay, Richard initially balked at the suggestion. But after considerable persuasion, he reluctantly agreed to follow Dr. Joseph's advice. Before long, he was accepting his medical degree from the Albert Einstein College of Medicine and moving on to a residency program in obstetrics and gynecology at the University of Michigan.

Upon completion of his residency in 1978, Dr. Walker relocated to Houston, Texas to begin his medical practice. Since then, he has changed his focus to integrative medicine, also known as orthomolecular medicine, in hopes of curing or preventing disease instead of merely managing it. This growing field integrates the best of traditional and alternative medical thought. He has also expanded into the fields of age management (anti-aging) and environmental medicine in his search for all possible approaches to therapy. According to the author, "people deserve the best there is available in healthcare."

Dr. Walker has served on the faculty of the University of Texas Medical Center, and is the founder and CEO of Walker Health Care Holdings and TVP-Care, LLC, Houston-based health companies. In addition to being a published writer, he is a highly sought-after speaker. The author attributes his remarkable and unlikely success to his wife, Marvia, who was the voice of encouragement and the force behind his achievement; his children, who, although they did not know the depth of his struggle, always said, "Dad, you can do it"; Professor Joseph, who saw something in him that he didn't know was there; and Major Ray Sumners, who was a guiding light to him throughout his time in the Air Force and was the person who taught him how to succeed.

Index

Black Broadway

African Americans on the Great White Way

Stewart F. Lane

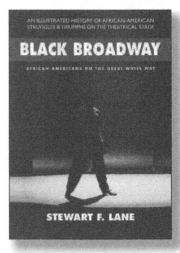

The Black actors and actresses whose names light up Broadway marquees have earned their place in history not only through hard work and talent, but also because of the legacy left by those who came before them. Like the doors of many professions, those of the theater world were shut to minorities for decades, and talented Black performers, playwrights, and musicians often had little opportunity to demonstrate their skills. It took men and women of determination to change the social landscape and open the theater doors not only to black artists, but to black audiences, as well. Here in this remarkable book is their stories beautifully told in words and illustrations.

$39.95 US • 288 pages • 9 x 12-inch hardback • ISBN 978-0-7570-0388-2

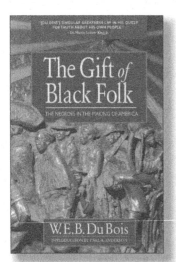

The Gift of Black Folk

The Negroes in the Making of America

W.E.B. Du Bois

A gifted writer, scholar, sociologist, historian, and activist, W.E.B. Du Bois was one of the founding fathers of the US Civil Rights movement. In 1924, during the height of the country's Black Renaissance, he produced a remarkable history of African-Americans— *The Gift of Black Folk.* This work represents one of the first insider's views of the Black experience in America. In it, Du Bois detailed the role of blacks in the early exploration of America; the roles they played in culti-vating tobacco, cotton, sweet potatoes, and peanuts; and the courage they displayed in fighting wars. He documented their creative genius in music, painting, sculpture, literature, theatre, and in virtually every aspect of American culture.

$14.95 • 288 pages • 6 x 9-inch quality paperback • ISBN 978-0-7570-0319-6

Your Blood Never Lies
How to Read a Blood Test for a Longer, Healthier Life
James B. LaValle, RPh, CCN

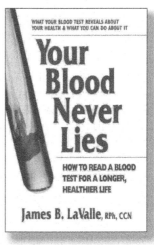

In *Your Blood Never Lies*, Dr. James LaValle clears the mystery surrounding blood test results. In simple language, he explains all of the information found on a typical lab report— the medical terminology, the numbers and percentages, and the laboratory jargon—and makes it understandable and accessible. This means that you can look at the test results yourself and understand the significance of each biological marker being measured. To help you take charge of your health, Dr. LaValle also recommends the most effective standard and complementary treatments for dealing with any problematic findings. Rounding out the book are explanations of lab values that do not appear on the standard blood test, but that should be requested for a more complete picture of health. A blood test can reveal so much about your body—and *Your Blood Never Lies* provides all the information you need to understand the results and take control of your health.

$16.95 US • 368 pages • 6 x 9-inch paperback • ISBN 978-0-7570-0350-9

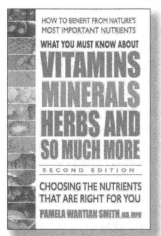

What You Must Know About Vitamins, Minerals, Herbs and So Much More • SECOND EDITION
Choosing the Nutrients That Are Right for You
Pamela Wartian Smith, MD, MPH

Now available in a fully revised edition that reflects the latest research and science-based studies, *What You Must Know About Vitamins, Minerals, Herbs and So Much More—Second Edition* explains how you can restore and maintain health through the wise use of nutrients. Part One of this easy-to-use guide presents the individual nutrients necessary for wellness. Part Two offers personalized nutritional programs for people with a wide variety of health concerns. People without prior medical problems can look to Part Three for their supplementation plans. Whether you are trying to overcome a medical condition or you simply want to preserve good health, this new Second Edition can guide you in making the best dietary and supplement choices for you and your family.

$16.95 US • 464 pages • 6 x 9-inch paperback • ISBN 978-0-7570-0471-1

WHAT YOU MUST KNOW SERIES

When it comes to your health, knowing the right thing to do is not always clear. Wading through the seemingly endless amount of information (and misinformation) on any health condition can be an exercise in frustration. The Square One "What You Need to Know About" series is here to help. Covering a wide range of topics, these titles, written by health professionals, provide everything you need to make informed decisions. Finding the right path to a healthier life is not always easy. Let this Square One series lead the way.

■ *What You Must Know About*
   STROKES
   $16.95 US • 320 pages •
   6- x 9-inch quality paperback •
   ISBN 978-0-7570-0483-4

■ *What You Must Know About*
   WOMEN'S HORMONES
   $17.95 US • 256 pages •
   6- x 9-inch quality paperback •
   ISBN 978-0-7570-0307-3

■ *What You Must Know About*
   THYROID DISORDERS
   $17.95 US • 256 pages •
   6- x 9-inch quality paperback •
   ISBN 978-0-7570-0307-3

■ *What You Must Know About*
   HASHIMOTO'S DISEASE
   $16.95 US • 272 pages •
   6- x 9-inch quality paperback •
   ISBN 978-0-7570-0475-9

■ *What You Should Know About*
   BIOIDENTICAL HORMONE
   REPLACEMENT THERAPY
   $17.95 US • 192 pages •
   6- x 9-inch quality paperback •
   ISBN 978-0-7570-0380-6

■ *What You Must Know About*
   LIVER DISEASE
   $17.95 US • 176 pages •
   6- x 9-inch quality paperback •
   ISBN 978-0-7570-0404-9

■ *What You Must Know About*
   DIALYSIS
   $17.95 US • 192 pages •
   6- x 9-inch quality paperback •
   ISBN 978-0-7570-0349-3

■ *What You Should Know About*
   DRY EYE
   $16.95 US • 144 pages •
   6- x 9-inch quality paperback •
   ISBN 978-0-7570-04479-7

■ *What You Must Know About*
   ALLERGY RELIEF
   $17.95 US • 224 pages •
   6- x 9-inch quality paperback •
   ISBN 978-0-7570-0437-7

■ *What You Should Know About*
   FOOD AND SUPPLEMENTS
   FOR OPTIMAL VISION CARE
   $16.95 US • 176 pages •
   6- x 9-inch quality paperback •
   ISBN 978-0-7570-0410-0

**For more information about our books,
visit our website at www.squareonepublishers.com**